Adult Physical Dysfunction and the Occupational Therapy Process

Tenika Danley, OTD

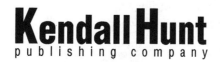

Kendall Hunt
publishing company

Cover image © Shutterstock, Inc.

Kendall Hunt
publishing company

www.kendallhunt.com
Send all inquiries to:
4050 Westmark Drive
Dubuque, IA   52004-1840

Copyright © 2021 by Kendall Hunt Publishing Company

ISBN 978-1-7924-7557-3

Printed in the United States of America

Table of Contents

Preface   *v*

Acknowledgments   *vii*

Contribution Author   *ix*

Section I   **Complete Occupational Therapy Evaluation**   **1**

CHAPTER 1   Occupational Therapy and the Occupational Therapy Process   3

CHAPTER 2   Visual Deficits   7

Section II   **Executive Function**   **15**

CHAPTER 3   Perceptual Dysfunction and Cognition   17

CHAPTER 4   Evidence-Based Occupational Therapy, Learning, Teaching, and Documentation   21

CHAPTER 5   Infection Control and Safety Issues in the Clinic   23

Section III   **Total Body Movement**   **27**

CHAPTER 6   Joint Movement and Measurement   29

CHAPTER 7   Motor Function and Occupational Therapy   35

Section IV   **Physical Debilitating Conditions**   **39**

CHAPTER 8   Cardiopulmonary Conditions and Occupational Therapy   41

CHAPTER 9   Sensory Dysfunction and Occupational Therapy   45

Section V   Orthopedic Conditions   49

CHAPTER 10   Orthopedic Conditions for the Upper and Lower Extremities   51

CHAPTER 11   Orthotics and Prosthetics   63

Section VI   Neurological Conditions   69

CHAPTER 12   Stroke and Occupational Therapy   71

CHAPTER 13   Traumatic Brain Injury   77

CHAPTER 14   Neurodegenerative Diseases of the Central Nervous System   83

Section VII   Spinal Cord Injuries   91

CHAPTER 15   Spinal Cord Injuries   93

Preface

This book was inspired by everyone in the world who has benefited from occupational therapy. Becoming an OT was the best decision I could have ever made. As occupational therapists we inspire, motivate, teach, and encourage those who need support. This book is dedicated to the students who made me fall in love with teaching and the clients who made me fall in love with occupational therapy. To my family and friends who have tirelessly supported me while completing this project. To my husband, thank you for your unwavering love, encouragement, and fantastic ideas! Finally, I want to give thanks to my Lord and savior, Jesus Christ, who has been my guide through it all. I am so very proud of this body of work, and it is my prayer that you are too.

Acknowledgments

I am so grateful to God for his everlasting mercy and grace for without him nothing is possible. To my husband who has been a constant support system and contributing author for this project. Farrish, I love you and I thank you from the bottom of my heart. To my mother, LaBrenda, you are truly the wind beneath my wings. You are a real-life example of living a purpose filled life. Ron, you have always been my role model for success and I still look up to you. To my family and friends, thank you all for the encouragement and laughs throughout this process. Writing this book has been a journey of strength, courage, and determination. I was pushed beyond my limits and though it was uncomfortable, difficult, and shed many tears, it is done. I love you all to no end and thank you!

Contributing Author

Farrish Danley, III, BS, MEd, EdS

Contributions were made to the following chapters:

Chapter 5:   Infection Control

Chapter 8:   Cardiopulmonary Function

Chapter 11: Orthotics

Chapter 15: Spinal Cord Injuries

SECTION I
Complete Occupational Therapy Evaluation

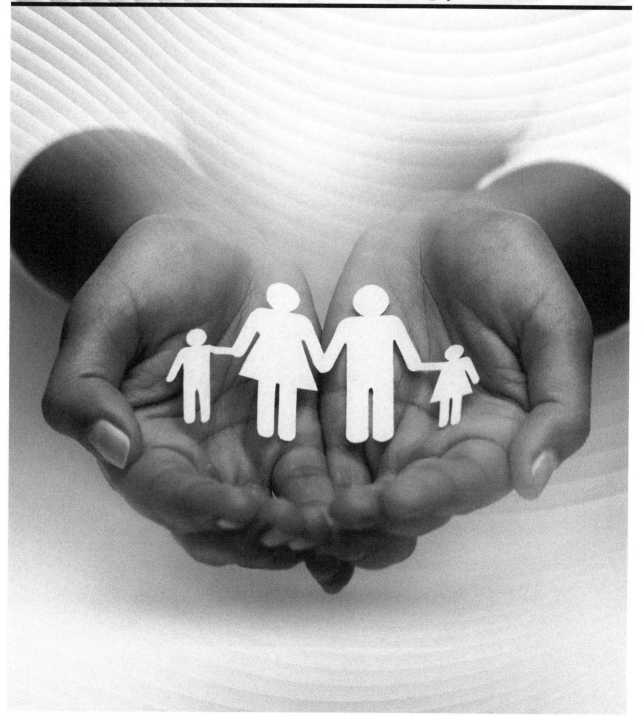

CHAPTER 1

Occupational Therapy and the Occupational Therapy Process

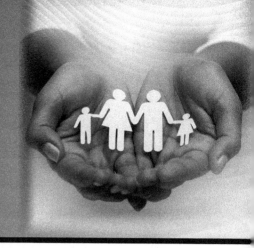

What Is Occupational Therapy?

Ever wonder what an Occupational Therapist does? Have you ever asked yourself what is Occupational Therapy (OT)? Occupational therapy is the use of a client-centered approach to improve the independent function of individuals or groups through active participation in meaningful activities. Everything we as occupational therapists do through activities of daily living (ADLs) contributes to the occupational therapy process and promotes quality of life (QOL). Therefore, when thinking of OT, consider a holistic approach. As OTs we treat the entire person cognitively, physically, and emotionally. OTs are dynamic, multifaceted clinicians, maximizing health and caring for the well-being of our clients.

Occupational therapy is the use of functional assessment and intervention to develop and maintain therapeutic use of self while completing ADLs through meaningful engagement in activity (AOTA, 2014). Occupational therapy is useful with groups, individuals, and communities to assist with the recovery process and improve functional independence (AOTA, 2014). Occupational therapy is a division of allied health and is performed by occupational therapists (OT) and certified occupational therapy assistants.

Occupational Therapy Process

The Occupational Therapy Practice Framework was developed to explain the legacy that occupational therapy has sustained for health promotion and engagement in occupation (AOTA, 2014). The occupational therapy process helps clients to attain preferred goals within his or her context and environments during participation in meaningful occupations (AOTA, 2014). The process includes evaluation and intervention to reach specific goals set by the OT and those goals also are components of the occupational therapy domain (AOTA, 2014). The domain is composed of five categories including (1) occupations, (2) client factors, (3) performance skills, (4) performance patterns, and (5) contexts and environments (AOTA, 2014). These areas of activity are also referenced as basic ADLs (AOTA, 2014).

During the OT process practitioners analyze activities and engagement in occupation while cooperating with the client to individualize intervention planning (AOTA, 2014). Occupational therapy practitioners use restoratively chosen occupations and activities as initial means of providing therapeutic intervention throughout the process (AOTA, 2014). The Occupational Therapy Framework is a fluid model designed to be adapted from single persons to groups, as necessary (AOTA, 2014). Whether OT intervention includes individuals or communities of people it must include information about the client's needs, wants, strengths, limitations, and occupational hazards, collectively, combined and outlined from an occupational therapy perspective (AOTA, 2014).

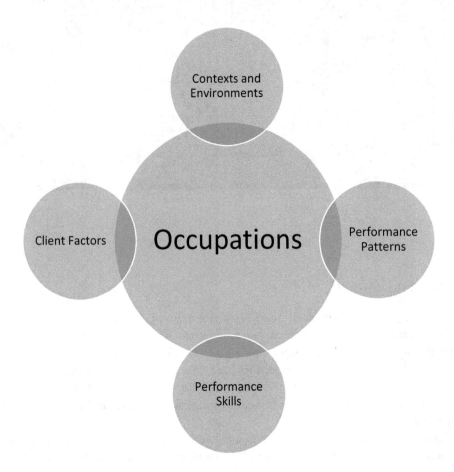

All aspects of the domain are interrelated and are of equal value, together they combine to affect the client's occupational identity, health, and well-being (AOTA, 2014).

Evaluation

The evaluation process is aimed at identifying what a client wants and needs to do, choosing what a client can do and has done and identifying factors for support as well as barriers to a healthy lifestyle (AOTA, 2014). Evaluation is an ongoing process and occurs during all interactions with the client (AOTA, 2014). All occupational therapy evaluations are client-centered and vary according to the treatment setting (AOTA, 2014).

The evaluation includes establishing an occupational profile and a breakdown of the client's occupational performance (AOTA, 2014). The occupational profile contains information regarding the client's deficits, needs, safety concerns, and performance of occupational tasks (AOTA, 2014). The occupational performance analysis highlights the client's limitations and strengths regarding occupational performance to focus on identified outcomes (AOTA, 2014).

Occupational Profile

The occupational profile is a compilation of the client's life experiences, habits and roles, occupational history, needs, preferences, and beliefs (AOTA, 2014). Establishing a client occupational profile provides the practitioner with insight into the client's point of view and environment (AOTA, 2014). A client-centered approach is most useful when gathering information for the occupational profile. Clients provide the most accurate information regarding personal beliefs, life goals, and meaningful occupations as it relates to the therapeutic intervention. When a practitioner places value on the client's ideals and needs it empowers the client and provides a sense of self-worth (AOTA, 2014). When the occupational profile is established using a client-centered approach the participation in daily activity should improve (AOTA, 2014). As the amount of time you spend with the client grows, the amount of information collected about the client should increase after a while (AOTA, 2014). There are different ways to collect information from clients including interviews, assessments, demonstrations, and observations. OT's ask questions like why this client is seeking services or what are the client's daily roles (AOTA, 2014). Once information-gathering has been completed the occupational therapist will develop a plan or a hypothesis for treatment based on the information that has been gathered up to this point in the therapeutic process. This plan for intervention is shaped around the specific deficits noted during information-gathering within the occupational profile (AOTA, 2014).

Intervention Process

During the intervention process occupational therapists use information gathered during the occupational profile to establish an intervention plan (AOTA, 2014). Therapists use theoretical principles to guide their occupation-based interventions (AOTA, 2014). Interventions are planned based on a client's ability to perform daily routines and roles of activity to engage in their lives. The client's ability to meet the physical, emotional, and cognitive demands of tasks will determine the type of occupational therapy intervention (AOTA, 2014).

The intervention process includes three phases: (1) intervention plan, (2) intervention implementation, and (3) intervention review (AOTA, 2014). It is during the intervention process that information is combined with evidence, models of practice, and theory to establish client-centered goals for each client (AOTA, 2014). The intervention plan directs the actions of occupational therapists and outlines specific occupational therapy approaches used throughout the intervention process to assist the client in attaining goals (AOTA, 2014). The design and details of the intervention plan and outcomes are aimed at attending to the client's current and possible scenarios related to participation in occupations (AOTA, 2014).

Intervention implementation is the process of acting out the intervention plan (AOTA, 2014). Intervention can either focus on one specific aspect of the domain or multiple aspects of the domain like performance skills and performance patterns (AOTA, 2014). Certain aspects of the domain influence one another in a fluid network so often that occupational therapist's expectation is to see clients modify, conform, and enhance in one area that will directly affect another area (AOTA, 2014). For this reason, the interconnectedness of the domains directly affects evaluation and intervention planning throughout the implementation process (AOTA, 2014).

The intervention review is the continuous process of reevaluating and reviewing the quality of the intervention plan's delivery and the client's need to achieve desired outcomes (AOTA, 2014). During this portion of the intervention process occupational therapists will partner with the client to discuss selected interventions based on the desired outcomes of the client (AOTA, 2014). It is during the intervention review that changes or modifications are made to the original intervention plan (AOTA, 2014).

Outcomes

Outcomes are the result of the occupational therapy process (AOTA, 2014). Outcomes describe what the client has achieved throughout the intervention process. Outcomes are related to the interventions provided by the occupational therapist and the domains related to the client's needs (AOTA, 2014). Outcomes are also related to the client's level of participation, physical ability, and perspective for attaining set goals (AOTA, 2014). Interventions can be designed for caregivers to improve both the QOL of the client and caregiver (AOTA, 2014). Outcomes for groups can include improved social interaction, better self-awareness via peer groups, a greater social network, and improved productivity in the workplace (AOTA, 2014). Outcomes are the focus throughout the occupational therapy process (AOTA, 2014).

National Board for Certification in Occupational Therapy (NBCOT) Domains

The National Board for Certification in Occupational Therapy has established its own set of domains to guide the occupational therapy evaluation and intervention process. This set of domains can be broken down into four categories. Those categories include (1) evaluation and assessment, (2) analysis and interpretation, (3) intervention management, and (4) competency and practice management (NBCOT, 2018).

In the first domain, evaluation and assessment, occupational therapists gather data related to traits that affect occupational performance throughout the occupational therapy process (NBCOT, 2018). The second domain involves the development of conclusion regarding the ideals and desires of the client to plan specific interventions throughout the occupational therapy process (NBCOT, 2018). The third domain refers to the intervention management specifically for guiding a client-centered plan throughout the occupational therapy process (NBCOT, 2018). The fourth and final domain involves competency and practice management of professional activities of self-care and related other tasks guided by evidence, practice standards, and regulatory agencies (NBCOT, 2018).

References

American Occupational Therapy Association. (2014). Occupational therapy practice framework: Domain and process (3rd ed.). *American Journal of Occupational Therapy, 68*(Suppl. 1): S1S48. http://dx.doi.org/10.5014/ajot.2014.682006

National Board for Certification in Occupational Therapy. (2018). Content Outline for the OTR Examination. https://www.nbcot.org

CHAPTER 2
Visual Deficits

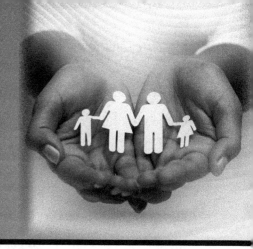

The ability to adapt to the environment and its surroundings requires the use of the visual system along with the integration of the visual stimulus via the retina to the brain. Visual perceptual processing can be organized in a hierarchy of processes and functions that contribute to one another (Warren, 1993). This hierarchy consists of visual cognition, visual memory, pattern recognition, visual scanning, and visual attention (Warren, 1993).

Neuroplasticity is the body's ability to adapt and interpret information via the nervous system and thus vision is an important component in our everyday learning. Visual skills are plastic in that they are repetitive skills that become more refined with frequent use (Pendleton & Schultz-Krohn, 1995). Vision is combined with other senses like touch, hearing, taste, and smell allowing us to interact with our environment in a more meaningful way.

There are three visual functions that comprise the foundation for all higher level visual and perceptual processing. Those functions are (1) oculomotor control, (2) visual acuity, and (3) visual field (Warren, 1993). Oculomotor control provides visual stability, visual acuity provides visual clarity—ability to see details, and visual fields provide awareness of objects and their surroundings (Warren, 1993). Without these baselines visual functions, accurate and pertinent information would not be generated in the CNS.

Glaucoma

Glaucoma is caused by increased ocular pressure which damages the peripheral retinal area by pushing against the optic nerve (Congdon, 2004; Fletcher, 1999). The clinical presentation reveals areas of the peripheral visual field that are obstructed, leaving the central visual field intact (Congdon, 2004; Fletcher, 1999). Medical treatment includes eye drops and surgery.

Macular Degeneration

Macular degeneration causes retinal scarring around the macula that impairs its function (Kahn, 1991). There is no known cause for macular degeneration but research indicates that the degeneration process is accelerated by UV rays (Kahn, 1991). The clinical presentation reveals deficits in the central visual field (Kahn, 1991). Medical treatment involves medication and laser surgery. The Amsler grid is used to detect signs of macular degeneration. A person who may be suffering from macular degeneration may see blurred lines on the grid or the lines may appear distorted. Other signs include the inability to focus on the black dot in the center of the grid.

Cataracts

Cataracts are a buildup of protein clumped in the lens of the eye and cause cloudy vision (Levin, 2004) (Rutner et al., 2006). The cause is trauma, diabetes, and the aging process. The process is accelerated by UV light. Medical treatment includes cataract-removal surgery.

Contrast Sensitivity

Contrast sensitivity describes the crispness of vision, enabling us to see objects that do not stand out from their backgrounds. Vision allows us to see things and process those things we see as light information. The yellow filter helps to improve contrast sensitivity. People presenting with signs of contrast sensitivity can have difficulty with seeing curbs and face recognition. The pupillary light reflex controls the diameter of the pupil.

Nystagmus

According to Pedretti, *nystagmus* is involuntary rhythmic shaking or wobbling of the eyes. There are two main types of acquired nystagmus: (1) *optokinetic* (*eye-related*) and (2) *vestibular* (*inner ear-related*). Nystagmus is caused by disease, accident, neurological problems, and medication. Medical treatment includes surgery, medication, and head-positioning techniques. The null zone is a position in which the nystagmus is least, and vision is best.

Low Vision versus Legal Blindness

Low vision is a visual impairment that cannot be corrected medically or surgically. The effects are severe enough to interfere with the performance of activities of daily living but do allow some vision. However, *legal blindness* implies any measure of vision loss from severe to total blindness. For a person to qualify as legally blind they must have a corrected visual acuity of 20/20 or less in the better eye or a visual field of 20 degrees or less in the better eye. Both low vision and legal blindness affect visual acuity which refers to the eye's ability to resolve detail to correctly identify information about a stimulus in space.

Visual acuity is measured using the standard Snellen eye chart with designations of 20/20, 20/30, 20/40, up to 20/200. The Snellen eye chart measures the person's ability to identify detail using letters, numbers, or figures of different sizes positioned on a chart 20 feet away. A score of 20/20 implies that a person's optical system is working properly.

Refractive Dysfunction

Myopia is nearsightedness and results in impaired distance vision while hyperopia or farsightedness results in impaired near vision. Significant degrees of farsightedness affect the ability to focus, therefore, causing blurred vision at both distant and near vision. *Astigmatisms* result in distortion of the visual image causing objects near and far to appear blurred.

Saccades

Saccades are rapid shifts of the eyes from object to object, allowing fast localization of movements in the periphery. Essentially, saccades are the eye's ability to change fixation from point to point. Saccades present clinically as skipping lines when reading or losing your place while reading. Some clients reread lines, words appear to hop around on the page, or experience letter order confusion. Other clients may experience poor hand-eye coordination and have difficulty with safety during mobility.

Visual Fields

The visual fields are created by a vertical line that bisects the face into a nasal and a temporal hemifield. The temporal half of the visual field is normally much larger than the nasal due to obstruction of the orbital margins and the nose. The visual field is the portion of space where objects can be perceived while the client is visually fixating on a single identified object located directly ahead but can also respond to targets peripheral to that specified object. Normal visual field reaches up to 135 degrees vertically and 160 degrees horizontally (Kandel & Wurtz, 2000). Visual field sensitivity is found the farther out the stimulus is from the center. Medical conditions that may present with visual field deficits include glaucoma, macular degeneration, diabetes, retinal detachment, and high blood pressure.

Visual Field Loss

Visual field loss is a physical loss of visual field to one side. Visual field loss presents clinically as running into objects, tripping, falling, knocking over drinks, and being startled by objects or people that suddenly appear in front of them. Signs and symptoms can also include difficulty reading and being fearful of falling. Clients can also become overwhelmed in crowds of people and develop associated problems like paralysis, cognition, ocular motor, or perceptual concerns.

Visual Neglect

Visual neglect is an attention deficit problem and clients are unable to attend to one side of their body. The client with both visual field loss and visual neglect has a worse prognosis for recovery than a client who presents with only one. The client will present with difficulty learning compensatory strategies.

Diplopia

Diplopia is double vision caused by dysfunction of the extraocular muscles, therefore, causing convergence insufficiency. *Strabismus* is a malalignment of the eyes where they do not point in the same direction. *Tropia* is a misalignment of the eyes when a client is looking with both eyes uncovered. *Phoria* is present when there is a break in the fusion of vision.

General Vision Assessment

A clinical vision assessment should be completed on all neurologically impaired patients as a part of a comprehensive neurorehabilitation program. The vision assessment helps to establish a baseline and quantifies the patient's visual performance. During the vision assessment you gather information regarding the patient's history, for example (1) Does the patient wear glasses? (2) Do they have prior visual impairments? Perform a chart review for optometry/ophthalmology reports for additional information.

Clinical Observation

During the clinical observation occupational therapists will watch how the eyes move together and individually. The OT will also observe how the eyes move in relation to the head and identify which activities are difficult for the patient. Other areas of observation include the patient's head position in relation to their trunk and asking the client to describe *what* they see or feel. Oculomotor assessment includes fixation, ocular alignment, range of motion, and smooth pursuits.

Performance and Function

During the performance and function occupational therapists will establish the patient's level of orientation. OTs will also establish a baseline for balance and the patient's ability to judge geographical areas. The occupational therapist will also determine the patient's rate of approach, safety concerns, and endurance levels. Other assessment considerations include environmental hazards, patient's position, cognitive function, communication ability, and fatigue.

Visual Acuity Intervention and Rehabilitation

The focus of visual rehabilitation is to identify and understand acuity problems to assist the client in performing activities of daily living. The focus strategy for visual rehabilitation is to improve the overall function of the visual system to allow the client to function at their highest level. Safety and education are important to discuss with the client regarding their visual deficits. Referral to an optometrist may be necessary if visual acuity deficits are identified during the assessment.

Visual acuity treatment intervention strategies are individualized for each client according to their deficits. Those interventions include proper eyewear, enlarged print, and improved contrast. Other considerations for visual acuity deficits can include minimizing the clutter in the client's environment, increased light with less glare (halogen or fluorescent), and bold tip pens.

Oculomotor Treatment Interventions

Oculomotor assessment includes observing the client's ability to look from one point to another or follow a moving object. Eye movement is a complex activity requiring coordination of eye muscles and rhythmic movement of the eyes together. Oculomotor dysfunction can be caused by a cerebral insult in the brain. Clinical signs and symptoms of oculomotor dysfunction can include the inability to function effectively and efficiently under prolonged near-point tasks. Other signs of oculomotor dysfunction include loss of place when reading or being easily distracted and slow when reading, as well as decreased reading comprehension. Clients may also experience headaches and eye fatigue or fluctuating depth perception. Vertigo, nausea, slowness to follow moving objects, omission of words, letter reversals, and word reversals are also signs of oculomotor dysfunction.

Other symptoms include the following:

- Inability to coordinate movement
- Diplopia
- Reduced figure-ground abilities (difficulty with details)
- Intermittent blurred vision
- Poor eye-hand coordination
- Poor eye movement
- Head tilt
- Close working distance
- Problems integrating inputs from other senses

Visual Fixation Treatment Interventions

Treatment intervention for visual fixation includes activities that encourage holding a gaze at an identified target. The goal during this intervention is to hold the gaze and not to move the eyes in another direction. To successfully complete fixation the client's attention must be intact. Other interventions include focusing on an object for a short period of time and then increasing the time. Begin with simple fixation and tabletop tasks, then move on to scanning and environmental attention to improve gaze stabilization.

Ocular Alignment and Range of Motion Treatment Interventions

A client can present with acquired or congenital ocular alignment deficits. If the deficit is due to muscle imbalance, then intervention can begin with exercise. Then incorporate task adaptation or modification of lifestyle. Medication and surgery are also treatments that can only be completed by a physician.

Saccades Treatment Interventions

Saccades treatment intervention can include puzzles, word search, newspaper cancellation therapies, last letter cancellation for right hemianopsia, wall fixation, and computerized trainers. Treatment for saccades also includes dyna-vision or similar training device, head and eye shifts, descriptive walking, post-it note hallways, search strategies, large table cards, or Wii tennis.

Visual Field Loss Treatment Interventions

Treatment intervention for visual field loss includes remedial and compensatory strategies. Remedial strategies address scanning exercises and compensatory strategies address independence. Other treatment interventions for visual field loss include client and family education to increase awareness. Treatment can also include referral to an eye care professional.

The remedial approach places objects on the affected side of the visual field, therefore forcing the client to look toward the affected side. The compensatory approach places objects on the unaffected side to increase independence. The compensatory approach can also include educating the client's family about visual field loss and how it may affect their loved one's function.

Diplopia Treatment Intervention

Treatment for diplopia can include patching one eye or active range of motion. Other treatments for diplopia can include prism, surgery, and botulinum toxin.

Please match the following terms with the correct definition listed below.

1. _____ Tracking

2. _____ Fixation

3. _____ Acuity

4. _____ Fusion

5. _____ Accomodation

6. _____ Ptosis

7. _____ Convergence

8. _____ Divergence

9. _____ Diplopia

10. _____ Strabismus

11. _____ Nystagmus

12. _____ Occlusion

13. _____ Binocular vision

14. _____ Monocular vision

15. _____ Temporal (anatomical direction)

16. _____ Nasal (anatomical direction)

17. _____ Optometrist

18. _____ Neuro-optometrist

19. _____ Ophthalmologist

20. _____ Neuro-ophthalmologist

a. drooping eyelid
b. clearly seeing
c. union of an image(s) into a single image
d. following a moving object
e. ability to adjust the distance it sees from
f. ability to maintain gaze
g. misalignment of the eyes
h. ability to turn eyes inward
i. double vision
j. ability to use the eyes as a team
k. Toward the nose, inward
l. Tremors of the eyes
m. Ability of both eyes to work together to focus, depth perception, and distance
n. Toward the temple, outward
o. To block out light
p. Ability of one eye to focus
q. Different stimuli of the retina are used to prevent confusion
r. Physician who specializes in disease affecting vision originating from the nervous system
s. Physician who specializes in eye and vision care
t. Healthcare professional who is licensed to provide primary eye care services
u. An optometrist who specializes in acquired visual dysfunctions

Define the following terms:

1. Hemianopsia
2. Saccades
3. Light sensitivity
4. Figure-ground
5. Visual memory
6. Visual discrimination
7. Visual closure
8. Spatial relationship
9. Agnosia
10. Neglect
11. Blind spot
12. Post-traumatic visual syndrome
13. Visual midline shift syndrome
14. Contrast sensitivity
15. Glaucoma
16. Macular degeneration
17. Cataracts

References

Congdon, N., O'Colmain, B., Klaver, C. C. W., Klein, R., Muñoz, B., Friedman, D. S., Kempen, J., Taylor, H. R., Mitchell, P., & Eye Diseases Prevalence Research Group (2004). Causes and prevalence of visual impairment among adults in the United States. *Archives of Ophthalmology*. 2004;122:477–485.

Fletcher, D. C., & Colenbrander, A. (2004). Introducing rehabilitation. In D. C. Fletcher(Ed.), *Low vision rehabilitation: Caring for the whole person* (monograph 12, pp 1–9). American Academy of Ophthalmology.

Kahn, J. (1991). Blunt trauma to orbital soft tissues. In B. J. Shingleton (Ed.). *Eye trauma*. Mosby.

Kandel, E., & Wurtz, R. (2000). Central visual pathways. In E. R., Kandel, J. H. Schwartz, & T. M. Jessell. *Principles of neural science* (4th ed.). McGraw-Hill.

Levin, L. L. (2004). Neuro-ophthalmologic diagnosis and therapy of central nervous system trauma. *Ophthalmology Clinics of North America, 17*, 455–464.

Pedretti, L. W., Pendleton, H. M. H., & Schultz-Krohn, W. (2013). Pedretti's occupational therapy: Practice skills for physical dysfunction (pp. 595, 597, 599, 600–602, 607, 611, 619). Mosby.

Pendleton, H. M., & Schultz-Krohn, W. (1995). *Pedretti's occupational therapy* (8th ed.). Mosby.

Rutner, D., Kapoor, N., Ciuffreda, K. J., Craig, S., Han, M. E., & Suchoff, I. B. (2006). Occurrence of ocular disease in traumatic brain injury in a selected sample: A retrospective analysis. *Brain Injury, 20*, 1079–1086.

Warren, M. (1993). A Hierarchical Model for Evaluation and Treatment of Visual Perceptual Dysfunction in Adult Acquired Brain Injury, Part 1. *American Journal of Occupational Therapy, 47*, 42–54. https://doi.org/10.5014/ajot.47.1.42

SECTION II
Executive Function

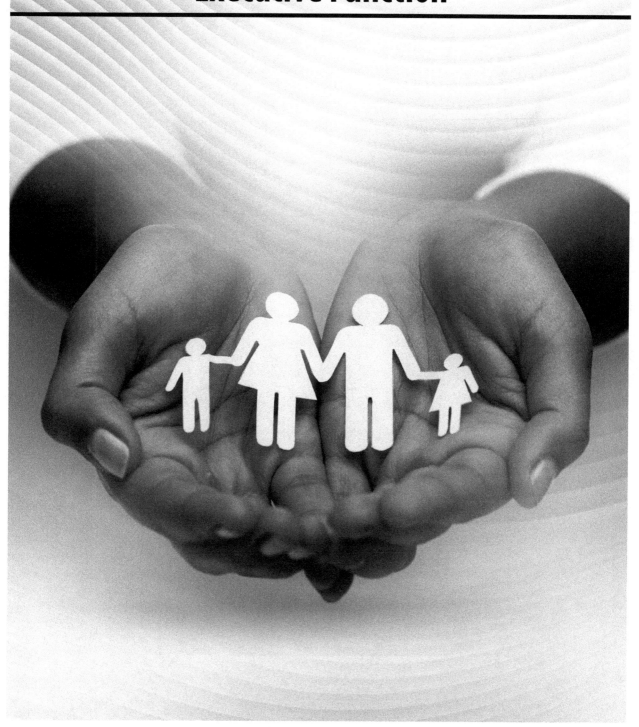

CHAPTER 3

Perceptual Dysfunction and Cognition

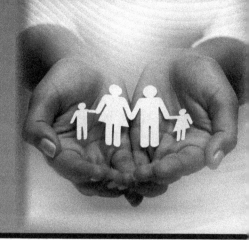

Visual perceptual disorders impair the client's ability to place meaning to visual data. When a visual perceptual disorder is present, a person's vision becomes undefined, and objects may be perceived as larger or smaller than their true size (Pedretti et al., 2018). Some clients also have trouble identifying colors and attaching meaning to various signs within their surroundings. Perception is the tool used by the brain to understand sensory stimuli received from the world around us (Pedretti et al., 2018). Perception is a learned processing skill for interpreting visual stimuli. Body scheme is the integration of all bodily systems working together to establish the foundation for all motor functions in the body (Ayres, 1972; MacDonald, 1960). Acquired visual perceptual deficits are usually found in people diagnosed with progressive neurological disorders (LeZak, 1995; Ogden, 1990).

Occupational Therapy Evaluation

Occupational therapy assessments include both verbal and motor responses including identifying an object verbally or completing a written task. A complete visual perceptual assessment allows for fluid responses for those clients with severe communication and cognitive limitations (Pedretti et al., 2018). Occupational therapists can use multiple assessments to evaluate clients to provide a thorough battery of data for review (Cooke et al., 2006). Monitoring the occupational performance and the perceptual-motor demands of functional tasks given to clients assist in the interpretation of information gathered during the assessment. A common method of assessment is the bottom-up approach, which breaks tasks down into small, separate parts of a client's skills (Warren, 1981; Warren, 1993a). The bottom-up approach can be used to assess visual clarity, eye muscle function, and several other basic visual skills necessary for refined visual processing.

Occupational Therapy Intervention

Adaptive approaches to intervention provide training in occupational therapy performance to facilitate client adaptation to specific contextual surroundings (Neistadt, 1990). Adaptive approaches use repetition or selected occupational performance tasks by providing alternative ways to compensate for deficits (Neistadt, 1990). While remedial approaches also called *transfer learning approaches* produce changes in the central nervous system, they hypothesize that several practice opportunities using a specific skill will generate subsequent use of the skill to like activities requiring the use of the same skill (Neistadt, 1990).

Evaluation and Intervention of Specific Perceptual Impairments

According to Pedretti, visual perceptual disorders inhibit a client's capacity to name and remember familiar items and individuals (Zoltan, 1996). People who have been diagnosed with agnosia are unable to visually describe items and orally communicate the identity of those items. Agnosia is often caused by the right occipital lobe or posterior multimodal association area (Humphreys & Riddoch, 1987; Lezak, 1995). Assessment of agnosia involves asking the client to recall five common items visually. If the client cannot identify four out of five items, then visual agnosia may be the cause (Pedretti et al., 2018). Color agnosia is the failure to recall and identify the unique colors of familiar items located in an area (Hécaen et al., 1956). Assessment includes identifying objects that are colored correctly versus the objects that are not colored correctly. Color anomia is a deficiency in the ability to identify the color of the items. Ask the client to name the color of various objects (Pedretti et al., 2018).

Metamorphopsia is a visual deformation of items like distinguishing the physical properties of size and weight (Zoltan, 1996). To assess metamorphopsia ask the client to place items in order by size or weight using only vision. Prosopagnosia is the failure to identify known faces due to injury of the right posterior hemisphere of the brain. The assessment for prosopagnosia is a face identification test that presents a variety of multiple choice and matching photos anteriorly and laterally under different lighting conditions (Benton & Fogel, 1962). Simultanagnosia is described as a deficit in determining and explaining a visual arrangement in its entirety and is due to injury to the right hemisphere of the brain (Ellis & Young, 1988). Ask the client to describe the details of an image and determine if the client can explain the entire scene.

Visual-Spatial Perception Disorders

Visual-spatial perception is described as the ability to value the structural organization of the body's anatomy in relation to oneself, and the connection between objects in space (Pedretti et al., 2018). The right hemisphere also controls dimensional abilities while the left focuses on distinct facts (Lezak, 1995). Figure-ground discrimination provides a person the ability to distinguish the foreground from the background in a variety of visual sequences (Pedretti et al., 2018). Form constancy is the identification of several constructs, shapes, and items, despite their orientation, placement, or size (Zoltan, 1996). Position in space is dependent on the locality of a shape or an object to oneself (Pedretti et al., 2018).

Right–Left Discrimination Dysfunction

The ability to correctly function under the constructs of right versus left is described as right–left discrimination (Zoltan, 1996). To assess right–left discrimination ask the client to identify different body parts and indicate if the body part is on the right side or left side. An alternative is to ask the client to follow verbal directions. Stereopsis describes as the lack of ability to sense depth in connection to different items in the area (Zoltan, 1996). Depth perception is essential to independently function in today's society. To assess depth perception, place assorted items in an area and ask the patient to determine which is closest and which is farthest away (Pedretti et al., 2018).

Tactile Perception Disorders

Individuals who are diagnosed with tactile perception disorders present with deficits in the second somatosensory area of the parietal lobes (Pedretti et al., 2018). Stereognosis, also known as tactile gnosis, (Dellon, 1981) is the technique that allows a client to recognize familiar items and structural shapes using touch without the use of vision. Astereognosis is described as the inability to identify objects without seeing them. Graphesthesia is best described by Pedretti as the ability to recall numbers, letters, or constructs written on the skin (Chusid, 1985; Geschwind, 1975). Body scheme perception disorders are defined as the inability to recognize their own body shape when the position becomes distorted (Pedretti et al., 2018). Finger agnosia is the incapacity to distinguish the fingers of the hand (Benton & Sivan, 1993).

Motor Perception Disorders

Pedretti states that praxis is the capability to specify and execute a meaningful movement. Apraxia is an impairment in the performance of acquired movement that is not explained by poor strength, lack of coordination, or decreased sensation, poor cognition or distractibility (Geschwind, 1975). Pedretti refers to three types of apraxia: (1) ideational apraxia, (2) ideomotor apraxia, (3) dressing apraxia. Ideational apraxia is the failure to use tangible items correctly (De Renzi, 1985; De Renzi et al., 1968; Haaland et al., 1999). Ideomotor apraxia is the decreased capacity

> **Learning Activity:**
>
> 1. Using an *adaptive approach* for treatment intervention.
> 2. Choose any perceptual deficit listed in the chapter.
> 3. List the problems associated with the deficit you chose.
> 4. Identify the evaluation and assessment tool (s).
> 5. Create an OT plan of care (goals).

to perform the motor requirements of a task using oral cues or simulation. Dressing apraxia is the decreased ability to effectively sequence motor actions required to perform upper and lower body dressing (Pedretti et al., 2018).

References

Ayres, A. J. (1972). *Sensory integration and learning disorders*. Western Psychological Services.

Benton, A. L., & Fogel, M. L. (1962). Three-dimensional constructional praxis: A clinical test. *Archives of Neurology, 7*(4), 347–354. doi:10.1001/archneur.1962.04210040099011

Benton, A. L., & Sivan, A. B. (1993). Disturbances of the body schema. In K. M. Heilman and E. Valenstein (Eds.) *Clinical neuropsychology*. Oxford University Press.

François, B., & Grafman, J. (2000). *Handbook of neuropsychology* (2nd ed., vol. 4). Elsevier.

Chusid, J. G. (1985). *Correlative neuroanatomy and functional neurology* (19th ed.). Lange Medical Publications.

Cooke, D. M., McKenna, K., Fleming, J., & Darnell, R. (2006). Criterion validity of the Occupational Therapy Adult Perceptual Screening Test (OT-APST). *Scandinavian Journal of Occupational Therapy, 13*(1), 38–48. doi:10.1080/11038120500363006

De Renzi, E. (1985). Methods of limb apraxia examination and their bearing on the interpretation of the disorder. *Advances in Psychology, 23*, 45–64. https://doi.org/10.1016/S0166-4115(08)61135-8. https://www.sciencedirect.com/science/article/pii/S0166411508611358

De Renzi, E., Pieczuro, A., & Vignolo, L. A. (1968). Ideational apraxia: A quantitative study. *Neuropsychologia, 6*(1), 41–52. https://doi.org/10.1016/0028-3932(68)90037-7. https://www.sciencedirect.com/science/article/pii/0028393268900377

Dellon, A. L. (1981). *Evaluation of sensibility and re-education of sensation in the hand*. Lippincott Williams & Wilkins.

Ellis, A. W., & Young, A. W. (1988). *Human cognitive neuropsychology*. Lawrence Erlbaum.

Geschwind, N. (1975). The apraxias: Neural mechanisms of disorders of learned movement. *American Scientist, 63*, 188.

Haaland, K. Y., Harrington, D. L., & Knight, R. T. (1999). Spatial deficits in ideomotor limb apraxia: A kinematic analysis of aiming movements. *Brain, 122*(6), 1169–1182. https://doi.org/10.1093/brain/122.6.1169

Hécaen, H., Penfield, W., Bertrand, C., & Malmo, R. (1956). The syndrome of apractognosia due to lesions of the minor cerebral hemisphere. *AMA Archives of Neurology & Psychiatry, 75*(4), 400–434. doi:10.1001/archneurpsyc.1956.02330220064007

Humphreys, G. W., & Riddoch, M. J. (Eds.). (1987). *Visual object processing: A cognitive neuropsychological approach* (1st ed.). Routledge. https://doi.org/10.4324/9781315456850

Lezak, M. D. (1995). *Neuropsychological assessment*. Oxford University Press.

MacDonald, J. (1960). An investigation of body scheme in adults with cerebral vascular accident. *American Journal of Occupational Therapy, 14*, 72.

Neistadt, M. E. (1990). A critical analysis of occupational therapy approaches for perceptual deficits in adults with brain injury. *American Journal of Occupational Therapy, 44*, 299.

Ogden, J. A. (1990). Spatial abilities and deficits in aging and age-related disorders. In F. Boller & J. Grafmans (Eds.), *Handbook of neuropsychology* (Vol. 4, pp. 265–278). Elsevier.

Pedretti, L. W., Pendleton, H. M. H., & Schultz-Krohn, W. (201i). *Pedretti's occupational therapy: Practice skills for physical dysfunction*. Elsevier.

Warren, M. (1981). Relationship of constructional apraXia and body scheme disorders to dressing performance in adult CVA. *American Journal of Occupational Therapy, 35*, 431–437.

Warren, M. (1993a). A hierarchical model for evaluation and treatment of visual perceptual dysfunction in adult acquired brain injury: part I. *American Journal of Occupational Therapy, 47,* 42.

Warren, M. (1993b). A hierarchical model for evaluation and treatment of visual perceptual dysfunction in adult acquired brain injury: part II. *American Journal of Occupational Therapy, 47,* 55.

Zoltan, B. (1996). *Vision, perception, and cognition* (3rd ed., (rev)). Slack.

CHAPTER 4

Evidence-Based Occupational Therapy, Learning, Teaching, and Documentation

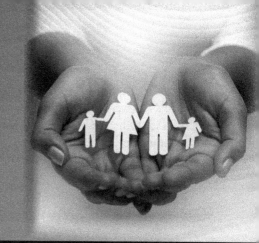

Systematic OT Practice

Systematic OT practice (SOTP) is a model that combines and builds on evidence-based approaches and how they relate to clinical practice. This model assists in the emergence of fresh OT information and its use clinically. This model is based on the evidence of current and related research findings.

There are three main sources of credible evidence used in evidence-based practice. They include client-generated sources, professional sources, and scientific evidence. Client-generated sources include patients and care-givers, professional sources include peers or other professionals, and scientific evidence includes research.

As occupational therapists we have made an ethical obligation to collaborate with clients regarding all aspects of their care, associated risks, and potential outcomes. As professionals we decide which ethical principles apply to each client, their situation, and why.

According to Pedretti, SOTP is the integration of critical analytic and scientific thinking with action processes throughout all phases and domains of OT practice. The integration of current and best evidence and the client's perspective are combined to guide the clinical reasoning process. The first phase of evidence-based practice is to select a theoretical framework to plan and assess the problem. Then evaluate the client, select interventions, identify desired outcomes, and create a plan of action. Evidence-based interventions are supported with research.

Evidence is the information used to justify a claim or a theory. This definition allows for the identification and acceptance of a larger scope of evidence as the foundation for clinical practice. Evidence is one of many reasons why SOTP is necessary. SOTP meets the service delivery demands of occupational therapy and provides a platform for expanded clinical practice. Another reason SOTP is essential to occupational therapy is to break through professional barriers via common language and ideas.

Inductive reasoning starts with information and ideas that are combined by their relationship to the information found during data collection. Common methods of inductive reasoning use interviews, observations, and textual context analyses (Pedretti et al., 2018). *Deductive reasoning* is a method used to break down the theory into separate components, which are then proven through testing. Common methods of deductive reasoning include samplings, measurements, and statistics (Pedretti et al., 2018). Problem statements identify a single theory regarding unwanted outcomes and decide what should be changed or modified. Problem mapping assists the OT in organizing the process of information-gathering to identify functional deficits with the client.

Teaching and Occupational Therapy

The purpose of teaching activities is varied for occupational therapy. Teaching activities assist clients in refreshing skills that were lost due to sickness or trauma. Teaching also helps clients integrate replacement or restorative techniques for performing meaningful tasks. Another purpose for teaching activities includes aiding clients in the development of new performance skills to support life roles as they relate to specific impairing diagnoses. Teaching activities provide therapeutic barriers for clients that will enhance performance skills to support aid in meaningful areas of occupation. One last purpose for teaching activities is to educate the clients' caregivers in tasks to improve the client's welfare and autonomy in daily occupation.

The principles of teaching occupational therapy can be applied to daily clinical practice in many ways. First you must determine a purposeful task for the client or family. Then you must choose an educational approach that blends with the traits of the task being learned. You must organize the instructional setting to provide support and grading of tasks with constructive criticism. Planned repetition through practice aids the client's learning process in daily function. The final principle of teaching a client is to develop self-reflection skills to enhance the carryover of learned tasks.

Learning and Occupational Therapy

There are three phases of learning: (1) acquisition phase, (2) retention phase, and (3) generalization phase. The acquisition phase happens within the first educational session with the student. Practice is often marked by multiple mistakes in task carryout as the student uncovers methods for achieving goals established in the intervention plan. The retention phase is evidenced by follow-up sessions when the student displays recall of the task in a familiar situation. The final phase of learning is the generalization phase also called the *transfer of learning* and is observed when the student can perform the learned task in different environments.

The two types of learning are procedural learning and declarative learning. **Procedural learning** is identified by the innate performance of tasks, lacking thought about how the task should be carried out. For example, learning to walk is procedural learning. Skills acquired through procedural learning are sharpened through repetition in a range of different contexts and environments (Pedretti et al., 2018). **Declarative learning** is the knowledge that is easily remembered. Skills learned through declarative learning usually require the use of memorization.

Case Study: Brian:

Brian sustained a closed head injury during a motor vehicle accident, resulting in cognitive deficits in attention, organization, and short-term memory. Before Brian's accident he worked as a clerk at the local library and was a full-time student majoring in engineering. Now Brian is unable to attend classes due to severe neck pain and fatigue, so he quit school and now works from home as a telemarketer. Brian uses neck pillows for support during work hours and uses a laptop computer. He takes rest breaks every 30 minutes and he is easily distracted, so completing household chores is impossible. Brian has recently been referred to OT.

1. Create a problem list.
2. Identify which Frame of Reference you will use.
3. Choose an intervention for each problem listed.
4. List two assessments that are appropriate for this client. Provide a brief description of each assessment and why it is applicable to this case. Be specific and provide details.

Reference

Pedretti, L. W., Pendleton, H. M. H., & Schultz-Krohn, W. (2018). *Pedretti's occupational therapy: Practice skills for physical dysfunction* (8th ed.). Elsevier.

CHAPTER 5

Infection Control and Safety Issues in the Clinic

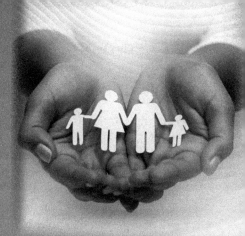

According to Pedretti, studies show that the environment in which OT services are provided directly affects the quality of services offered to the client. Providing a clean and safe environment for service delivery offers a feeling of comfort and improves the client's confidence in the clinician's competence. Infection control procedures are incorporated in the medical field to prevent the spread of contagious diseases among patients, healthcare clinicians, and the surrounding community. Infection control procedures were developed to establish a defense against the spreading cycle of disease. Universal precautions were designed to protect healthcare workers and the patients for whom they provide service from spreading diseases, such as viruses or bacterial infections.

The Centers for Disease Control and Prevention established specific infection control guidelines according to the method of transmission for pathogens and other infectious agents. **Body substance isolation** alienates wet or damp and possibly infectious substances from all patients. These agents include feces, urine, sputum, saliva, wound drainage, and other bodily fluids (Pedretti et al., 2018). **Standard Precautions** combine the main features of Body Substance Isolation and Universal Precautions (Pedretti et al., 2018). Standard Precautions apply to all bodily fluids including non-intact skin, mucous membranes (mouths, rectum, vagina), fluids, and blood. Transmission-based precautions are additional standard precautions which require the use of two methods of prevention for infectious pathogens. The first step is the defense from the infectious agent the client is carrying, and the second is the enactment of supplemental procedures to contain the spread of the infectious agent.

Occupational Safety and Health Administration (OSHA)

Occupational Safety and Health Administration (OSHA) is the regulatory body for healthcare providers such as hospitals and nursing homes. OSHA is a federal agency that creates and enforces national workplace safety standards. OSHA's mission is to ensure that all men and women in the US workforce have safe and healthful working conditions (The Balance Small Business, 2021). Each facility has a coordinator who conducts quarterly training sessions on how to access and treat a hazard in the facility. For example, they will be instructed on how to contain a spill and how to isolate a person who has been exposed to risk. This can have a huge impact on the ability to control the spread of infectious diseases in the workplace. To reduce the worker exposure to potential occupational hazards, including biologic agents, there needs to be feasible and effective measures that can be implemented in the workplace. Teach the staff basic practices to prevent the spread of infectious diseases. OSHA is responsible for the following guidelines:

- Educating employees on methods of transmission and prevention.
- Providing acceptable protective equipment and teaching employees where equipment is housed in the facility.
- Providing satisfactory containers for the disposal of sharps, waste, and other hazardous materials.
- Posting warning labels and biohazard signs.
- Providing education and follow-up care to employees who have been exposed to infectious disease.

Transmission-Based Precautions

According to CDC guidelines there are three types of transmission-based precautions used in healthcare today (CDC, 2007). Those precautions are contact precautions, droplet precautions, and airborne precautions. **Contact precautions** help prevent the transmission of infectious agents that are spread by direct or indirect contact with polluted areas or infected people. Contact Precautions are in effect when specific organisms pose a threat of transmission. Clients are placed in isolation when the presence of infectious disease has been confirmed through testing. When contact precautions are in effect personal protective equipment (PPE) must be worn to decrease the risk of exposure. Examples of PPE are gowns, gloves, foot and eye protection, protective hearing devices, hard hats, respirators, and full-body suits (Pedretti et al., 2018). Gloves should be worn any time there is a risk for contact with bodily fluids. Gloves must be changed between clients.

Droplet precautions prevent the transmission of pathogens spread through mucous membrane contact via respiratory secretions. Respiratory secretions include secretions via coughing, sneezing, and talking. Droplet precautions protocol consists of room isolation, respiratory PPE, and limited movement or transfer of the client unless the movement is necessary. **Airborne precautions** prevent the transmission of infectious organisms that remain suspended in the air over long distances. Airborne precautions include room isolation and masks (Pedretti et al., 2018).

According to Pedretti, an infectious disease often refers to the transmittable spread of pathogens from one person to another in varied ways. Preventing the spread of infectious disease requires basic infection control procedures including the appropriate hand-washing technique, contact precautions, and a clean workplace. The greatest mode of transmission for infectious diseases is via the hands. Therefore, it is crucial for healthcare professionals to use alcohol-based hand gels and anti-bacterial soap to cleanse the hands as often as possible to reduce the transmission of infectious diseases.

According to the CDC, the COVID-19 virus is thought to be spread mainly from person to person who are in close contact with one another (Centers for Disease Control, Retrieval date March 7, 2021). Respiratory droplets produced when an infected person coughs, sneezes, or talks can land in the mouths or noses of people who are nearby or possibly be inhaled into the lungs. Masks should be worn to prevent inhalation of droplets. Airborne transmission occurs when small droplets and particles travel farther than six feet and linger in the air after a person has left the space. Surface contamination can also spread the COVID-19 virus. The virus can be spread if a person places their hands on an infected area and touches their mouth, eyes, and nose. Hand washing is especially important. It is the single most effective means of preventing the spread of any infectious disease. Hands should be washed with soap and water for 20 seconds. Hand sanitizer should be used if soap and water are not available. Habitually clean and disinfect commonly touched areas and avoid crowded places (Website: https://www.cdc.gov/coronavirus/2019-ncov/prevent-getting-sick/how-covid-spreads.html

Disinfection and cleaning the facility are vital to maintain a safe working environment. For example, staff will wear face masks and wash their hands frequently. Next, disinfect all touch points, not just the frequently touched surfaces. Remove any visible soil with a cleaner before applying a disinfectant. Disinfect surfaces from clean areas to dirty areas. Specifically, restroom should be cleaned last because it is highly contaminated (Website: https://www.cdc.gov/coronavirus/2019-ncov/community/disinfecting-building-facility.html?CDC_AA_refVal= https%3A%2F%2Fwww.cdc.gov%2Fcoronavirus%2F2019-ncov%2Fcommunity%2Forganizations%2Fcleaning-disinfection.html Disinfection of Facility (March 7, 2021)

Emergency Considerations

- Cardiopulmonary resuscitation (CPR) training is a requirement for occupational therapists. The American Heart Association and the American Red Cross are both agencies that provide this certification for healthcare professionals.
- Fall risks are present in the clinical setting when functional mobility is included in the plan of care for clients. Safety measures to decrease the risk for falls include ensuring the therapeutic environment is clear of excess debris and equipment. Occupational therapists should use WC, gait belts, and remain in close proximity to clients who are participating in dynamic activities.
- Burns are usually minimal and first-degree and should be treated with basic first aid protocols.

- Bleeding is usually present as a result of a cut or an injury. To treat a bleed in the OT clinic apply basic first aid procedures using a new dressing.
- Shock occurs as a result of a hemorrhage, an infection, and a breathing difficulty. Shock creates a significant drop in blood pressure and poor cardiac output. Clients become pale, sweat abnormally, and are breathing inefficiently.
- Seizures are due to injuries to the brain and medication. Clinical presentation for seizures includes rigidity that lasts for a short time and then strong jerky motions follow.
- Insulin-related illnesses occur because a client has significantly lower insulin levels, abnormally high blood glucose levels (hyperglycemia), or abnormally low blood glucose levels (hypoglycemia). Ketoacidosis also known as hyperglycemia and hypoglycemia (insulin shock or insulin reaction) can both cause levels of unconsciousness requiring medical treatment. Insulin shock is due to an overload of insulin in a person's system, the lack of food or sugar, or over-exertion of muscles. Hyperglycemia is caused by decreased insulin levels or alters an individualized food regimen issued by a doctor. Usually, insulin injection is necessary to treat hyperglycemia, do not give these patients any sugar.
- Respiratory distress is present when a person is having difficulty breathing due to an obstructed airway. Dyspnea control postures alleviate shortness of breath for patients in respiratory distress. High Fowler's position is used for clients who are in bed. High Fowler's requires the head of the bed to be raised at 90 degrees. The orthopneic position is best described as a patient leaning forward on a stable surface bearing weight through their arms. Pursed lip breathing is another intervention used to address respiratory distress. Pursed lip breathing is performed by holding the lips together as if you were drinking from a straw and breathing in through the nose, then exhaling through the small hole in the lips. This technique increases airway resistance, therefore, dilating the constricted airways allowing for improved breathing.

References

Centers for Disease Control and Prevention, Healthcare Infection Control Practices Advisory Committee. (2007). *2007 guideline for isolation precautions: preventing transmission of infectious agents in healthcare settings, US Department of Health and Human Services, Centers for Disease Control.* http://www.cdc.gov/hicpac/pdf/isolation/Isolation2007.pdf

COVID-19. (March 7, 2021). https://www.cdc.gov/coronavirus/2019-ncov/prevent-getting-sick/how-covid-spreads.html

Disinfection of Facility. (March 7, 2021). https://www.cdc.gov/coronavirus/2019-ncov/community/disinfecting-building-facility.html?CDC_AA_refVal=https%3A%2F%2Fwww.cdc.gov%2Fcoronavirus%2F2019-ncov%2Fcommunity%2Forganizations%2Fcleaning-disinfection.html

Pedretti, L. W., Pendleton, H. M. H., & Schultz-Krohn, W. (2018). *Pedretti's occupational therapy: Practice skills for physical dysfunction* (8th ed.). Elsevier.

The Balance Small Business. (February 15, 2021). What is OSHA? Retrieved from https://www.thebalancesmb.com/what-is-the-occupational-safety-and-health-administration-osha-5092188

SECTION III
Total Body Movement

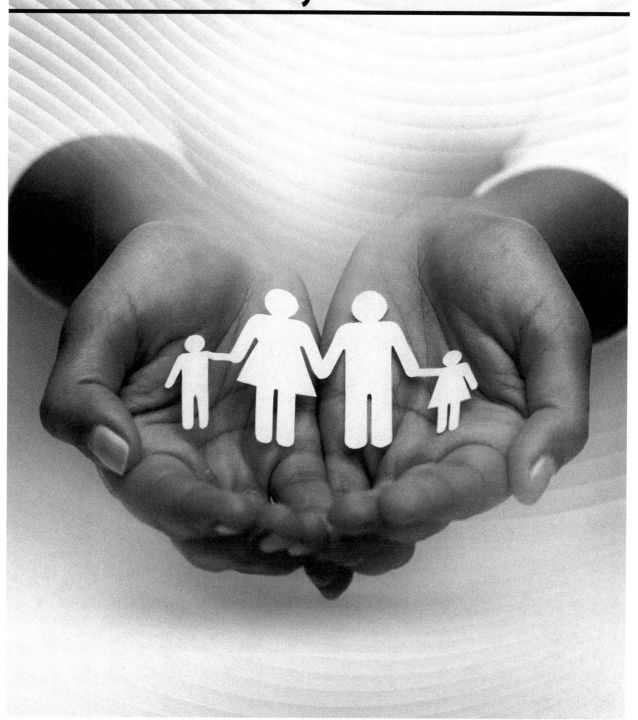

CHAPTER 6

Joint Movement and Measurement

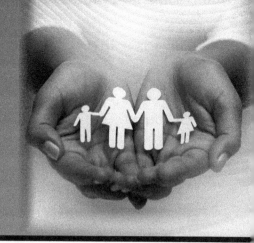

Joint measurement is important to occupational therapy to determine limitations that interfere with function or may produce deformity. Joint measurement is the amount of motion available at a joint (Brunnstrom, 1970). It is especially important to measure joint mobility to establish a baseline for documentation. It is also important to assess specific conditions and limitations that affect the range of motion. Joint measurement is used in many other areas to assist therapists in identifying strategies to reduce limitations. Examples of disabilities that can cause limited joint motion include stroke, traumatic brain injury, trauma, and neurodegenerative diseases.

When measuring joint range of motion, it is important to review the OT Practice Framework III in the areas of occupation, performance skills, and client factors. Occupations are any area of life that the client views as important including life roles or routines. Performance skills address motor performance and client factors address body functions including cognition, sensation, neuromusculoskeletal, cardiovascular, speech, and skin. Any of these areas of occupation can impact a client's joint mobility. The first step in joint measurement is to assess the mobility or range of motion of the joint through observation. Limited joint ROM can be due to spastic muscles, weakness, edema, and pain (Cole et al., 1988; Kendall et al., 2005).

Assessment tools include observations and interviews for gathering data regarding the daily performance of activities of daily living. Evaluation, re-assessment, and discharge are all components of the data-gathering process for joint measurement. Assessment is an ongoing process and should continue with each client visit.

Types of Range of Motion

Joint ROM is defined as the amount of movement that is possible at a given joint. There are four types of joint ROM: (1) active, (2) passive, (3) functional, and (4) active-assistive ROM (AAROM). Active ROM (AROM) is present when a joint is moved by the muscles that act on the joint. Passive ROM is present when a joint is moved by an outside force such as a therapist. PROM is greater than AROM secondary to the stretch of connective tissue (Brunnstrom, 1970; Daniels & Worthingham, 1986). Functional ROM is the amount of joint range necessary to perform essential ADLs and IADLs without the use of equipment. Active-assistive ROM is defined as ROM that is either initiated or completed by an outside force.

Joint Measurement Protocol

Joint measurement is performed to establish a baseline for joint range of motion, joint structure, and function. Joint measurement is also important in determining an end-feel, positioning, and identifying bony landmarks (Brunnstrom, 1970, 1972). During joint measurement occupational therapists should be capable of the following: visual observation, palpation, optimal therapist position, client limb support, and precautions or contradictions associated with the client's joint mobility (Daniels & Worthingham, 1986).

Occupational therapists should position themselves in a manner that is conducive for joint measurement and stabilization. Observe the joint for muscle deformity, discoloration, and skin integrity (3). Palpation is necessary to identify bony prominences for correct goniometry placement (3). During the final component of joint measurement, the occupational therapist moves the joint through its range of motion and assesses the movement for an estimate.

Before completing a full range of motion assessment with a client, a range of motion screen can be done to gather client data. During the range of motion screen, you first assess the joint for pain and limitations of the use of the joint. Next, you assess AROM at the therapist's direction and then PROM. During the PROM portion of the screen, you assess for end-feel, which is the normal resistance to continue joint motion due to stretching. Be sure to pay attention to the needs of your client when assessing ROM.

Goniometer Components

The goniometer has three components: the body, stationary arm, and moveable arm (Brunnstrom, 1970; Daniels & Worthingham, 1986). The body is the large round part of the goniometer with numbers listed around the edge for reading measurements. The stationary arm is always closest to the client and does not move for joint measurement. The moveable arm lies parallel to the stationary arm and moves follow the circumference of the body of the goniometer for joint measurement. Proper goniometer placement is essential to obtain accurate joint measurements to assist with intervention planning.

One Hundred- and Eighty-Degree System (180)

The starting point for the 180-degree system is zero (Brunnstrom, 1970; Daniels & Worthingham, 1986). Next, you move the goniometer toward 180 degrees to obtain the measurement (Brunnstrom, 1970; Daniels & Worthingham, 1986). When using the 180-degree method of measurement, hyperextension is noted with a (+) and extension limitations are noted with a (–). This measurement system is most used among occupational therapists. Most motions are measured with the client in anatomical position.

Contraindications for Joint Measurement

- Joint dislocation
- Unhealed fracture
- Immediately after surgery to soft tissue structures around the joint
- Ectopic ossification

Precautions for Joint Measurement

- Joint inflammation
- Infection
- Osteoporosis
- Hemophilia
- Hematoma
- Recent injury to soft tissue surrounding the joint
- Newly united fracture
- Prolonged immobilization
- Carcinoma (Brunnstrom, 1970; Crepeau et al., 2008)

Conditions that affect joint mobility

AROM is an intervention for scaring because it provides internal stretch against resistant scar tissue and cannot be overused. Range of motion can help control edema and assist with tendon gliding. Skin contractures like adhesions or scar tissue can limit the range of motion. Bony obstructions can also be hindrances to joint mobility. Spasticity, weakness, pain, and/or edema can also affect functional mobility of joints and limit use.

Several scenarios can produce a deficit associated with a limited range of motion. Some of those deficits present as soft tissue damage, joint trauma, and joint immobilization. Inflexibility at the joint can also affect strength and the speed of movement. Any of these deficits can impact a client's performance and quality of movement.

Intervention Planning for Joint Measurement

Occupational therapists analyze the results of the ROM screen as it relates to the client's life roles and habits. The focus is to improve the client's functional levels and increase any ROM that is limiting their performance of ADLs, self-care, and home maintenance. Methods to increase ROM include stretching, resistive exercise, strengthening, activities that require AROM, splints, and joint mobilization with modalities. Compensatory techniques can be used if the loss of ROM is permanent.

Manual Muscle Test

A manual muscle test (MMT) is defined as evaluating the maximal contraction of a muscle or muscle group (Clarkson, 2000; Clarkson & Gilewich, 1989). Contraindications of MMT include pain, inflammation in the joint being tested, dislocation, unhealed fracture, recent surgery, and bone carcinoma. Fragile bone disease can also be considered a contraindication for MMT.

The purpose of MMT is to determine the amount of power available in a muscle or group of muscles. MMT can also establish a baseline for the intervention of muscle weakness limiting a client's performance (Killingsworth, 1987). MMT assists occupational therapists with preventing deformities and identifying assistive devices. Other implications for MMT are to identify how muscle weakness is limiting occupation and to identify the need for assistive devices (Killingsworth, 1987). Screen tests are completed to identify which muscle groups require specific MMT (Clarkson, 2000; Daniels & Worthingham, 1986; Hilsop & Montgomery, 1995; Pact et al., 1984). Screens are completed by observing a client during the performance of a functional activity.

The Standard Procedure for measuring MMT ensures accuracy and consistency of data collection. The following steps comprise the Standard Procedure: (1) Position, (2) Stabilize, (3) Palpate, (4) Observe, (5) Resist, (6) Grade. Provide clear instructions to the client and ensure the correct position to prevent muscle substitutions during measurement. Undetected muscle substitutions can mask the client's problem and result in incorrect intervention planning. MMT limitations include a lack of measurement of muscle endurance, muscle coordination, and substitutions.

Muscle Grades

Muscle grades are documented using a scale from 0 to 5 with 0 being no muscle contraction and 5 being maximal resistance. There is a total of 10 levels within the 0 to 5 scale. A score of 0 (zero) constitutes no muscle contraction and a score of one (trace) constitutes contraction without movement. Gravity minimized position can assist with MMT for incomplete ranges of motion which are demonstrated in scores of 2– to 2+ (10, 14,). Muscle grades against gravity include 3– to 3, which can also indicate an incomplete range of motion. Complete ROM against gravity describes muscle grades from 3+ to 5 all performed with resistance. To assess MMT effectively and accurately, occupational therapists must have the knowledge, clinical reasoning skills, and experience.

Assessment for Intervention Planning

Occupational therapists use the results of the strength assessment to determine the progression of the intervention plan. The results of the MMT are also used to identify the degree of weakness and whether the weakness is specific to one or more muscles. MMT findings can determine if there is any difference in the muscle grades on each side including the agonist and antagonist muscles. Occupational therapists must also determine the client's level of endurance and implement compensatory strategies when necessary.

Measurement of Grasp and Pinch

There are two types of functional grasp: mature and immature. A mature grasp looks like a three-jaw chuck and an immature grasp looks like a fist. It is important for occupational therapists to identify which grasp is more functional for the client to complete self-care tasks. In addition to the two grasps, there are three types of pinch: (1) tip pinch, (2) lateral pinch, and (3) palmar pinch or three-jaw chuck. The tip pinch can best be described as pad-to-pad contact. The lateral pinch is best described as the thumb placed superior-laterally to the index finger, like turning a key in a lock. The palmar pinch can be described as the index and middle finger placed superiorly to the thumb, which is adducted and inferior.

References

Brunnstrom, S. (1970). *Movement therapy in hemiplegia*. Harper & Row.

Brunnstrom, S. (1972). *Clinical kinesiology*. F. A. Davis.

Clarkson, H. M. (2000). *Musculoskeletal assessment* (2nd ed.). Lippincott Williams & Wilkins.

Clarkson, H. M., & Gilewich, G. B. (1989). *Musculoskeletal assessment*. Lippincott Williams & Wilkins.

Cole, J. H., Furness, A. L., & Twomey, L. T. (1988). *Muscles in action*. Churchill Livingstone.

Crepeau, E. B., Cohn, E. S., & Schell, B. A. (2008). *Willard and Spackman's occupational therapy* (11th ed.). Lippincott Williams & Wilkins.

Daniels, L., & Worthingham, C. (1986). *Muscle testing* (5th ed.). W. B. Saunders.

Hislop, H. J., & Montgomery, J. (1995). *Daniels and Worthingham's muscle testing* (6th ed.). W. B. Saunders.

Kendall, F., McCreary, E. K., Provance, P. G., Rodgers, M., & Romani, W. (2005). *Muscles: Testing and function with posture and pain* (5th ed.). Lippincott Williams & Wilkins.

Killingsworth, A. (1987). *Basic physical disability procedures*. Maple Press.

Pact, V., Sirotkin-Roses, M., & Beatus, J. (1984). *The muscle testing handbook*. Little, Brown.

Matching

1. _____ Screening test

2. _____ Against gravity

3. _____ Gravity minimized

4. _____ Muscle endurance

5. _____ Resistance

6. _____ Substitutions

7. _____ Muscle coordination

a. Muscle or group of muscles compensate for function of a weaker muscle for movement
b. Movement that is parallel to the floor
c. Smooth rhythmic interaction of muscle function
d. Determines areas for specific MMT
e. Number of times the muscle can contract at its max level
f. Movement away from flow of blood

Define the following:

1. Muscle grade 0:

2. Muscle grade 1:

3. Muscle grade 2(–):

4. Muscle grade 2:

5. Muscle grade 2(+):

6. Muscle grade 3(–):

7. Muscle grade 3(+):

8. Muscle grade 4(–):

9. Muscle grade 4:

10. Muscle grade 4(+):

11. Muscle grade 5:

CHAPTER 7

Motor Function and Occupational Therapy

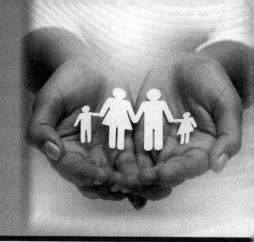

According to Pedretti, motor control is simply the central nervous system (CNS) organizing and controlling the body's participation in meaningful activity via muscles (Pedretti et al., 2018). Components of the CNS involved in motor control include the cerebral cortex, basal ganglia, and cerebellum. Pedretti also states that neuroplasticity is brain's ability to regenerate after damage. Upper motor neurons (UMN) are composed of the cell bodies that originate from the spinal cord and anatomy closest to the spinal cord. The anatomy of the UMN is made up of the brainstem, descending tracts of the spinal cord, and brain cells. UMN presents clinical signs and symptoms such as hyper-reflexia, positive Babinski sign, and spasticity. Other symptoms of UMN effects appear as weakness, paralysis, and fatigue. Lower motor neurons are located in the anterior horn cells of the spinal nerves. Lower motor neuron abnormalities present as decreased deep tendon reflexes and muscle weakness, atrophy, and flaccidity. Guillain-Barré is a lower motor neuron disease.

Assessment for Motor Control

Occupational therapy assessments for motor control should always be client-centered like the following:

- The Canadian Occupational Performance Measure (COPM; Law et al., 1998)
- The Stroke Impact Scale (http://www.pattersonmedical.com)
- The Stroke Specific Quality of Life Scale (Williams, 1999)

Standardized occupational therapy assessments should be completed according to the instruction provided. Examples of standardized assessments include the following:

- The Graded Wolf Motor Function Test (Morris et al., 2002)
- The Fugl-Meyer Assessment (Katz et al., 1992)
- The Assessments of Motor Process Skills (AMPS; Bernspång & Fisher, 1995)
- The Wolf Motor Function Test (Allergan, n.d.)

Muscle Tone

Muscle tone is described as the opposition of the muscle being assessed as the tester moves the extremity through the range of motion (Shumway-Cook & Woollacott, 2007). When a normal muscle is stretched passively, there is little involuntary opposition. Normal muscle tone is also dependent upon a functioning CNS and stretch reflex. Abnormal tone presents clinically as:

- Flaccidity—no tone; deep tendon reflexes are inactive.
- Hypotonus—low tone; deep tendon reflexes are minimal.
- Hypertonus—increased tone.

- Cerebral hypertonia—variations in muscle tone in flexion or extension for long periods of time, due to TBI, stroke, anoxia, neoplasms, cerebral palsy, metabolic disorders, brain diseases.
- Spinal hypertonia—immediately follows flaccid tone phase of a spinal cord injury and develops flexor tone, then extensor tone due to spinal stenosis, tumor.
- Spasticity—increased tonic reflexes identified by excessive tendon spasms, with subsequently increased excitability of the stretch reflex (Nance & Ethans, 2011) (a component of UMN function).
- Clasp-Knife—the clinician moves the limb through a fast passive stretch, resulting in an abrupt catch or opposition, followed by a reduction of the opposition.
- Clonus—present with moderate spasticity; repeated contractions in the antagonist muscles in reaction to quick stretch. Common in the finger and ankle flexors.
- Rigidity—combined increase in muscle tone of the agonist and antagonist; not velocity-dependent and is present following TBI, Parkinson's disease, degenerative diseases, and tumors. Can be present following carbon monoxide poisoning or ingestion of toxins. There are four types of rigidity:
- Lead pipe—steady opposition throughout the ROM, when the limb is moved gradually in a given plane, common in Parkinson's disease.
- Cogwheel—submission of muscle tone after regular, rhythmic opposition; common in Parkinson's disease.
- Decorticate—flexion rigidity of the upper limbs and extension of the lower limbs.
- Decerebrate—rigid extension posture in all four limbs and the neck.

Seizures and Todd's paralysis must be identified through differential diagnosis because the clinical presentation is very similar to CVA. The occupational therapy intervention for Todd's paralysis and seizures differs from that of a CVA.

Assessment of Muscle Tone

Tone assessment is completed by first ensuring the client is seated with their weight is distributed equally throughout the hips and trunk (Ryerson, 2007). Hold the client's extremity that is to be tested just distal to the joint being assessed and move it gradually through the available range of motion. Next secure the limb on the sides to prevent tactile stimulation of the muscle belly. To assess spasticity the clinician takes the extremity being tested and moves it quickly through the available range of motion. Rigidity is assessed by moving the extremity being tested through the available range of motion slowly. Be sure to list any opposition or resistance identified during assessment.

Measurement Scale for Tone

The Modified Ashworth Scale and Ashworth Scale are both tools that are commonly used during tone measurement for occupational therapists (Ashworth, 1964). Conflicting evidence exists regarding the validity of both scales use for measuring spasticity (Allison et al., 1996; Blackburn et al., 2002; Bohannon & Smith, 1987; Farrell et al., 2007; Gregson et al., 1999, 2000). The Ashworth Scale ranges from 0 to 4, with 0 being no increase in muscle tone and 4 is limb rigidity in flexion or extension (Ashworth, 1964).

Normal Posture Mechanics

The normal postural mechanism is made up of the innate mobility that develops as a result of dependable movements made by the body. Automatic functions occur very early during the developmental process and continue throughout development. These postural developments present clinically as righting reactions, equilibrium reactions, and protective reactions. Righting reaction is described as the ability to maintain the head in an upright position. Equilibrium reaction assists a client in keeping a position. Protective reactions are incorporated to prevent falls and loss of balance (FOOSH injuries). Assessment for righting reactions can be completed during functional activities and mobility. Equilibrium and protective reactions can be assessed during weight shifting tasks and lower body ADL completion (Pedretti et al., 2018).

Primitive Reflexes

According to Pedretti, brainstem level reflexes include asymmetric tonic neck reflex (ATNR), which is tested with the client seated or supine. The stimulus is passively or actively turning the client's head 90 degrees to either side. The response presents clinically as increased extensor tone in bilateral limbs on the facial aspect and increased flexor tone on the back of the head. The symmetric tonic neck reflex (STNR) is tested with the client seated or on all four extremities. The stimulus is flexing the client's head, bringing the chin to the chest. The response presents clinically as flexion in the upper limbs and extension of the lower limbs. The tonic labyrinthine reflex (TLR) is tested with a client supine with the client's head in the midline position. The stimulus is testing position. The response presents as an increase in flexor or extensor tone in the limbs. The positive supporting reaction is tested when pressure is applied to the ball of the foot. The stimulus is the pressure on the ball of the foot. The response presents as an increase in rigid extension of the lower extremities.

Spinal-Level Reflexes

Pedretti states that spinal reflexes occur as a result of a UMN injury. Amplified spinal reflexes include deep tendon reflexes, Babinski sign, flexor withdrawal, crossed extension, and grasp reflexes (Jain et al., 1995). Crossed extension reflex presents clinically as increased extension tone in one leg while the other is flexed. This reflexive pattern impairs functional mobility. Flexor withdrawal reflex presents with the ankle in a flexed position, as well as the knee and hip when the ball of the foot is stimulated through touch. This reflexive pattern impairs functional mobility including transfers. The grasp reflex is present when an object placed in the hand cannot be released.

Coordination

Coordination is the potential to supply correct, meticulous movement. Traits of coordination include uniformed, continuous movements, performed with the correct speed, and requiring fewer muscle groups to execute the movement. Appropriate posture, tone, and muscle tension are all required to produce coordinated movements. Incoordination is any disruption of coordinated movement secondary to the injury of the cerebellum. Cerebellar disorders present clinically as:

- ataxia
- dysdiadochokinesis
- dysmetria
- asynergia
- nystagmus
- dysarthria

Incoordination disorders can also be caused by the damage to the extrapyramidal cells of the brain. These disorders present clinically as:

- chorea
- athetoid movements
- dystonia
- ballism
- tremors—action, resting, essential (inherited)

Occupational Therapy Intervention

OT intervention is varied as it pertains to a motor control intervention. Weight-bearing improves motor unit facilitation in the upper limbs (Brouwer & Ambury, 1994). Motor cortical activity and prehension grasp for kids have also shown improvement through weight-bearing in the upper extremity. The recruitment of more afferent fibers is a result of the input from bearing weight (Chakerian & Larson, 1993). Proprioceptive neuromuscular facilitation (PNF) is helpful in improving motor control (Ryerson, 2007). Assessment using neuro-developmental treatment (NDT; Howle, 2002) as intervention includes the following:

- Complete a detailed functional movement evaluation
- Modify the environment in which the tasks are performed
- Educate the client about abnormal movement and compensatory techniques

Casting inhibits abnormal postures and reduces muscle tone. Casting a client in inhibitory postures produces reductions in tone and postures due to placing the joint in a neutral position, warmth from the cast material, constant pressure, and consistent muscle stretching. Physical agent modalities (PAMS) can be used to prepare or in addition to meaningful activity including muscle re-education. Hot, cold, ultrasound, and NMES are all examples of PAMS that can assist in the facilitation of motor control by increasing tendon and muscle excitability. Nerve blocks are medication prescribed by and inserted by a physician.

References

Allergan. (n.d.). *Botox package insert* [Allergan Pharmaceuticals]. http://www.allergan.com

Allison, S. C., Abraham, L. D., & Petersen, C. L. (1996). Reliability of the Modified Ashworth Scale in the assessment of plantar-flexor muscle spasticity in patients with traumatic brain injury. *International Journal of Rehabilitation Research, 19*, 67–78.

Ashworth, B. (1964). Preliminary trial of carisoprodol in multiple sclerosis. *Practitioner, 192*, 540–542.

Bernspång, B., & Fisher, A. G. (1995). Differences between persons with right or left CVA on the Assessment of Motor and Process Skills. *Archives of Physical Medicine and Rehabilitation, 76*, 1114–1151.

Blackburn, M., van Vliet, P., & Mockett, S. P. (2002). Reliability of measurements obtained with the Modified Ashworth Scale in the lower extremity of people with stroke. *Physical Therapy, 82*, 25–34.

Bohannon, R. W., & Smith, M. B. (1987). Interrater reliability of a Modified Ashworth Scale of muscle spasticity. *Physical Therapy, 67*, 206–207.

Brouwer, B. J., & Ambury, P. (1994). Upper extremity weight-bearing effect on corticospinal excitability following stroke. *Archives of Physical Medicine and Rehabilitation, 75*, 861–866.

Chakerian, D. L., & Larson, M. A. (1993). Effects of upper-extremity weight bearing on hand-opening and prehension patterns in children with cerebral palsy. *Developmental Medicine & Child Neurology, 35*, 216–229.

Farrell, J. F., Hoffman, H. B., Snyder, J. L., Giuliani, C. A., & Bohannon, R. W. (2007). Orthotic aided training of the paretic limb in chronic stroke: Results of a phase 1 trial. *Neurorehabilitation, 22*, 99–103.

Gregson, J. M., Leathley, M. J., Moore, A. P., Smith, T. L., Sharma, A. K., & Watkins, C. L. (2000). Reliability of measurements of muscle tone and muscle powering in stroke patients. *Age Ageing, 29*, 223–228.

Gregson, J. M., Leathley, M., Moore, A. P., Sharma, A. K., Smith, T. L., & Watkins, C. L.. (1999). Reliability of the Tone Assessment Scale and the Modified Ashworth Scale as clinical tools for assessing poststroke spasticity. *Archives of Physical Medicine and Rehabilitation, 80*, 1013–1016.

Howle, J. M. (2002). *Neurodevelopmental treatment approach: Theoretical foundations and principles of clinical practice.* Neuro-Developmental Treatment Association.

Jain, N., Florence, S. L., & Kaas, J. H. (1995). Limits on plasticity in somatosensory cortex of adult rats: Hindlimb cortex is not reactivated after dorsal column section. *Journal of Neurophysiology, 73*, 1537–1546.

Katz, R. T., Rovai, G. P., Brait, C., & Rymer, W. Z. (1992). Objective quantification of spastic hypertonia: Correlation with clinical findings. *Archives of Physical Medicine and Rehabilitation, 73*, 339–347.

Law, M., Baptiste, S., Carswell, A., McColl, M. A., Polatajko, H., & Pollock, N. (1998). *Canadian occupational performance measure* (3rd ed.). Canadian Association of Occupational Therapists.

Morris, D. M., et al. (2002). *Graded wolf motor function test* (revised). University of Alabama.

Nance, P. W., & Ethans, K. (2011). Spasticity management. In R. L. Braddom, L. Chan, M. A. Harrast, K. J. Kowalske, D. J. Matthews, K. T. Rangarsson, & K. A. Stolp (Eds.), *Physical medicine and rehabilitation* (4th ed., pp. 641–659). Elsevier/Saunders.

Pedretti, L. W., Pendleton, H. M. H., & Schultz-Krohn, W. (2018). *Pedretti's occupational therapy: Practice skills for physical dysfunction* (8th ed.). Elsevier.

Ryerson, S. D. (2007). Hemiplegia. In D. A. Umphred (Ed.), *Neurological rehabilitation* (5th ed.). Elsevier/Mosby.

Shumway-Cook, A., & Woollacott, M. H. (2007). Constraints on motor control: An overview of neurological impairments. In A. Shumway-Cook & M. H. Woollacott (Eds.), *Motor control: Translating research into clinical practice* (3rd ed.). Lippincott Williams & Wilkins.

Williams, L. S. (1999). Development of a Stroke Specific Quality of Life Scale. *Stroke, 30*, 1362–1369.

SECTION IV
Physical Debilitating Conditions

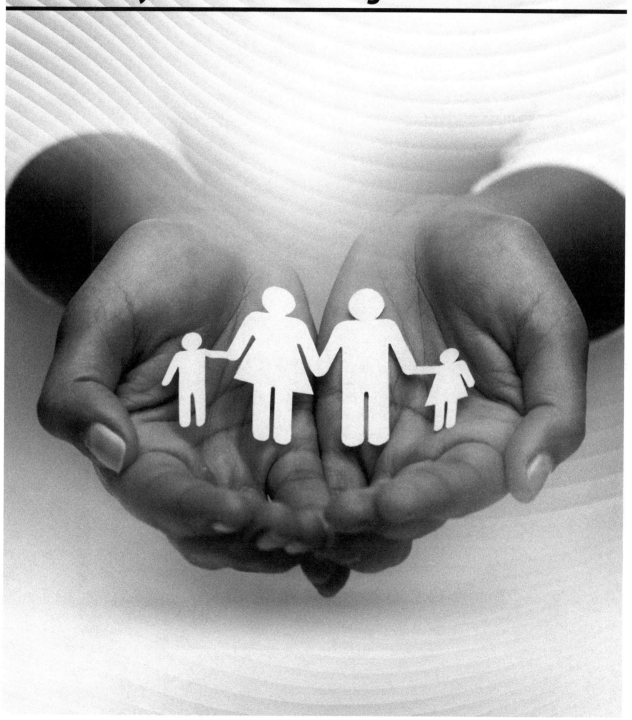

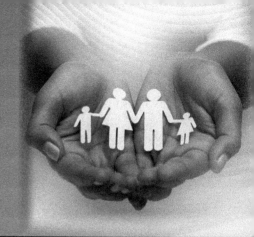

CHAPTER 8
Cardiopulmonary Conditions and Occupational Therapy

Cardiopulmonary conditions are the number one killer of women in the United States alone. Heart disease killed almost 400,000 women in 2017—or about 1 in every 5 female deaths (American Heart Association, 2018). Controllable risk factors for heart disease include smoking, high-lipid counts, increased cholesterol, high blood pressure (hypertension), sedentary lifestyle, diabetes, stress, and being overweight (AOTA, 2013). Uncontrollable risk factors include family history, age, and sex (AOTA, 2013).

Heart disease can be caused by a blocked coronary artery or anatomical anomalies of the heart. Ischemic heart disease can develop when portions of the heart temporarily lack oxygen. The most notable cause for ischemic heart disease is coronary artery disease and it is the most prevalent form of heart disease in the United States. **Coronary artery disease** is present when the coronary arteries are blocked or appear decreased in width, therefore are unable to efficiently perfuse the heart. CAD is most often caused by atherosclerosis, which is the buildup of cholesterol and increased fatty deposits on the inner lining surface of the artery. According to Pedretti, CAD is initially treated surgically via percutaneous transluminal coronary angioplasty (PTCA) or coronary artery bypass graft (CABG). Pacemakers provide an electrical shock to the heart muscle and adjust the heart rate to a normal pace. According to Pedretti, pacemakers are used to treat irregular heart rhythms called arrhythmias.

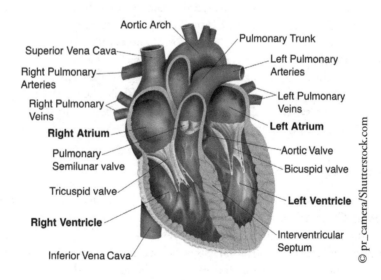

Cardiac Precautions (Sternal Precautions)

Pedretti states that following cardiac precautions following surgical intervention promotes the safest and most effective manner of intervention for occupational therapy clients. Cardiac precautions include the following:

- Precautions last up to 8 weeks following surgery
- Clients should avoid quick UB movement

- Avoid lifting anything over 8 lb.
- No pushing or pulling
- No driving
- Wear compression garments on the legs
- Hold a pillow to the chest when coughing or sneezing
- Inform the doctor if you hear a pop or click

Heart Disease Classification

According to the American Heart Association there are four categories of heart disease based on the metabolic equivalent rate or MET. Basic metabolic equivalent rates are equal to 3.5 ml oxygen per kilogram of body weight per minute (Ainsworth et al., 2000).

Class I—no physical limits in place and no complaints.
   MAX MET level is 6.5

Class II—minimal activity limits, comfortable at rest, common activity causes fatigue, shortness of breath, pain, and increased heart rate.
   MAX MET level is 4.5

Class III—Noted increase in physical limits, more comfortable at rest, marked fatigue, shortness of breath, and chest pain.
   MAX MET level is 3.0

Class IV—Unable to perform physical activity without discomfort, cardiac insufficiency may be present.
   MAX MET level is 1.5

Cardiac Diseases

Common heart diagnoses that are commonly treated by occupational therapists are myocardial infarction (MI), coronary artery disease (CAD), congestive heart failure (CHF), and cardiomyopathies (AOTA, 2013). Other diagnoses include acute coronary syndrome and angina pectoris. The **acute coronary syndrome** is caused by a rapid reduction in the blood perfusion to the heart and can progress to a heart attack if it is not treated. **Angina pectoris** is heart pain due to poor perfusion of the heart tissue. **Congestive heart failure** is present when the pumping action of the heart is unable to adequately perfuse the heart to satisfy the body's needs. Right-side heart failure is due to poor blood supply from the systemic circulation to the heart muscle from the right ventricle. Left-side heart failure is caused by the inability of the left ventricle to adequately remove blood from the lungs.

Valvular Heart Disease

Heart valves control blood flow direction as it travels through the heart. If damage occurs to the heart muscle blood flow will decrease. Complications like volume or pressure overload and aortic stenosis can lead to less than adequate perfusion of the systemic circulation. **Volume overload** is a buildup of fluid in the lungs causing dyspnea. Volume overload can be due to a faulty mitral valve that fails to close correctly. Blood is pushed back into the atria as the left ventricle is contracting. **Atrial fibrillation** is also the result of defects in the contractions of the atria. **Aortic stenosis** is present when the width of the aorta becomes narrow, resulting in pressure overload that causes the left ventricle to work harder. The left ventricle increases in size and lowers cardiac output. Resulting diagnoses can include the following:

- Ventricular arrhythmia
- Cerebral insufficiency
- Syncope
- Death

Myocardial Infarction

The heart tissue is formed in three layers: epicardium, myocardium, and endocardium. The epicardium is the inner layer of the pericardium. The myocardium is the largest part of the heart. The endocardium is the smooth lining of the inner surface and heart cavities, while the pericardium is the fibrous protective sac enclosing the heart. Myocardial infarction (MI) is caused by death or damage to the heart muscle due to poor perfusion. Heart attacks can present with several complications including the following:

- Inflammation of the pericardium
- Tears in the heart muscle
- Blood clots
- Aneurysms
- Heart failure
- Death

Transmural MI (STEMI) is the deadliest type of heart attack and involves all three layers of the heart. Non-ST elevation MI (NSTEMI) is due to a dangerously narrowed artery without completely blocking the coronary artery. An anterior MI (AWMI) results from left anterior descending artery damage due to blockage. The inferior MI (IWMI) is due to the obstruction of the right coronary which causes damage to the left ventricle.

Cardiac Rehabilitation

Phase I—monitor electrocardiogram (ECG), blood pressure, and pulse; assess for changes in the diagnosis; use the MET levels to assess ADL performance and other activities; observe for endurance and activity tolerance; home exercise program with adaptations for task simplification, activity guidelines, and risk factors (AOTA, 2013).

Phase II—Participate in skilled OT up to 3 days per week for 8 weeks; adjust activity according to the MET levels; education regarding risk factors; assess for psychosocial concerns and work hardening.

Phase III—community rehab; requires a physician's referral; stress test; and continued activity from phase II with less supervision.

Chronic Lung Disease

According to Pedretti, **chronic obstructive pulmonary disease** (COPD) is damage to the alveolar walls and inflammation of the conducting airway. COPD has two main diagnoses: emphysema and chronic bronchitis. Emphysema is due to gradual damage to the alveoli and chronic bronchitis is due to inflammation of the bronchial airways causing excess mucous production that blocks the airways. Smoking is the leading cause of COPD. COPD makes it difficult to breathe and causes coughing that produces wheezing and dyspnea. Physiological causes for COPD include the following:

- Airways and sac lose elasticity.
- The walls between the sacs are destroyed.
- The airways become thicker and inflamed.
- Increased mucous production clogs the airways.

There are four stages of COPD ranging from mild to very severe COPD. The mild stage begins with a chronic cough and mucous production. The moderate stage presents a chronic cough with increased mucous production and dyspnea. The severe stage of COPD presents with a chronic cough, increased mucous production, and fatigue. The last and most severe stage of COPD is the stage four marked with chronic cough, increased mucous production, severe dyspnea, changes in skin color, and weight loss. Asthma is a chronic lung disease that is present due to an inflamed and narrow airway.

Pulmonary Rehabilitation

The goal of pulmonary rehabilitation is to evaluate ADL performance to improve functional endurance and to provide instruction on breathing techniques for ADL completion. Assessing UE strength and adjusting the workload through task simplification or energy conservation is key in pulmonary rehabilitation. Occupational therapists can recommend adaptive equipment or adapt leisure activities to assist the client through the rehab process. Providing education for clients regarding stress management and relaxation techniques is also important during pulmonary rehab. Occupational therapy intervention involves ADL evaluation and training, breathing techniques like pursed-lip breathing and diaphragmatic breathing, and UB function. Evaluation should include monitoring heart rate and blood pressure following participation in activity.

References

American Heart Association. (2018). https://www.heart.org/-/media/files/about-us/policy-research/fact-sheets/access-to-care/cvd-womens-no-1-health-threat-fact-sheet.pdf?la=en

American Occupational Therapy Association. (2013). AOTA's NBCOT Exam Prep: Cardiopulmonary Condition.

Ainsworth, B. E., B. Sternpeld, M. T. Richardson, and K. Jackson. (2000). Evaluation of the Kaiser Physical Activity Survey in Women. *Medicine & Science in Sports & Exercise, 32*(Suppl.).

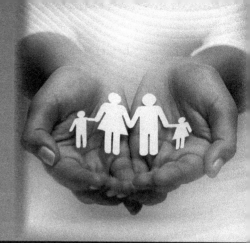

CHAPTER 9
Sensory Dysfunction and Occupational Therapy

Neural reorganization occurs in three phases which are habituation, learning and memory formation, and cellular recovery. These phases occur in order to allow the brain to form and identify synaptic connections after an injury called neuroplasticity. Neuroplasticity is directly affected by sensory perception and receptor morphology. The somatosensory system manages sensory input from the superficial sources or deeper sources of the body (Malaviya, 2003). Sensory receptors are specialized to react to specific kinds of stimuli. Mechanoreceptors respond to touch, pressure, stretch, and vibration. Chemoreceptors respond to injury or damage that have been stimulated by the release of chemical material. Thermoreceptors respond to hot or cold stimuli and nociceptors respond to pain. Nociceptors respond to painful stimuli (Lundy-Ekman, 2007).

Dermatomes

According to Pedretti, dermatomes are areas of skin that are supported by a single spinal root and the attached nerve. Dermatomes assist with sensory mapping along central lesions only. Dermatomes and spinal cord level correlate with the level of the lesion. Damage to peripheral nerves will follow a different pattern of innervation secondary to regrouping of the axons throughout the brachial plexus. Sensation deficits as a result of damage to central or peripheral lesions present as paresthesia, hyperalgesia, dysesthesia, and allodynia. Paresthesia feels like small bugs crawling or pins and needles. Hyperalgesia is heightened pain usually happens during nerve repair. Dysesthesia is an uncomfortable nerve sensation as a result of stimulation. Allodynia presents as pain sensitivity from a non-painful stimulus. Neuropathy is a sensory dysfunction due to nerve damage in the peripheral nervous system. Sensation is lost in a specific order as follows:

- discriminative touch
- proprioception
- cold
- hot
- pain

Superficial Sensation

Pedretti states that superficial sensation includes touch, pain, and temperature and are all identified as cutaneous sensation. Touch includes pressure and vibration which are stimulated by touch receptors. Touch receptors are organized into categories superficial, subcutaneous, coarse, temperature, and pain receptors. Superficial fine touch receptors include Meissner's corpuscles which respond to light touch and vibration, and Merkel's disks which respond to pressure. Subcutaneous fine touch receptors include Pacinian corpuscles which respond to touch and vibration, and Ruffini's corpuscles which respond to skin stretching. Coarse touch receptors respond to rough or uncomfortable touch. Temperature receptors called C-fibers respond to heat stimulus, and A-delta fibers respond

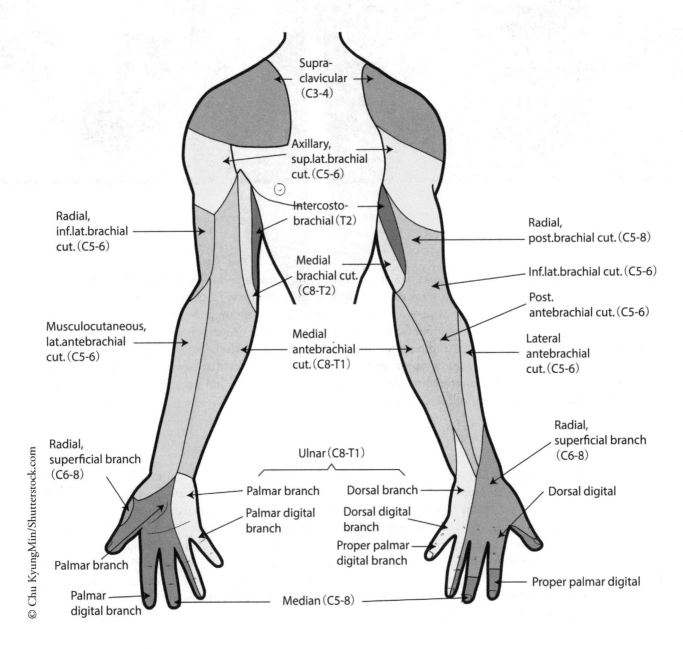

to cold stimulus. The final category of superficial sensory receptors is pain receptors that respond to irritated nerve endings due to cellular injury secondary to edema.

Sensory Topography

According to Pedretti, proprioception is the awareness of joint's position in space. Proprioception is essential to the connection between cortical and cerebellar pathways to define motor planning and adaptation. The sensory arrangement of the cerebral cortex allows information regarding the identity and location of sensory input to be transmitted through communication pathways in the brain. This sensory input is then processed in the brain as touch, proprioception, pain, and temperature. Discriminative touch, the body's position in space, and identifying objects without the use of vision are examples of sensory input that is communicated through a 3-neuron pathway in the brain. This 3-neuron pathway consists of receptors to the medulla, medulla to the thalamus, and thalamus to the cerebral cortex. Next, information is obtained and categorized in the primary somatosensory cortex. The homunculus can be used to identify the location and function of many sensory receptors in the body.

Evaluation

A sensory evaluation requires attention to detail, accuracy, and a proper client environment. To begin you must establish a quiet and therapeutic experience for the client. Then, you ensure that your tools are in place and you understand the components of the sensory evaluation. Next, you obstruct the client's vision and provide clear, concise instructions for the client to follow. Providing a calm environment for the client allows them to relax and participate fully during the evaluation process (Pedretti et al., 2018).

Assessment

During the assessment phase for sensory function occupational therapists gather additional information about the client including hand dominance, grip or pinch strength, motor function, the time that the injury occurred, and the nature of the injury. Pedretti states that the sympathetic phenomena can be described as sympathetic and cutaneous sensory fibers continuing along the same pathway, and the sympathetic involvement becomes more dominant due to the median nerve makeup. For this reason, Complex Regional Pain Syndrome is more prevalent in clients who have been diagnosed with median nerve injuries. Keeping in mind that there are more sympathetic nerve fibers in the upper extremity, assessing involuntary responses as they relate to sensory function is very important during the sensory assessment. Occupational therapists should look for skin blotching, abnormal sweat response, lack of erector pili muscle function, and fingertip atrophy (Pedretti et al., 2018).

Mapping Sensation

According to Pedretti, sensory mapping allows a client to identify places of deficit on the hand before the initial test is administered. The sensory innervation of the hand is composed of the ulnar nerve, radial nerve, and median nerve. The dorsum and palm both contain superficial cutaneous branches of the median, ulnar, and radial nerves. The Semmes-Weinstein monofilament can be used to assess sensory function on the unaffected side first. After you have assessed the sensory function on the affected side perform the same test on the unaffected side for comparison (Pedretti et al., 2018).

Sensation Screen

According to Pedretti, median nerve screening begins at the thumb, tip, index tip, and index proximal phalanx. Ulnar nerve screening starts distally and moves proximally at the little finger and the proximal ulnar palm. Screening for the radial nerve occurs in the webspace of the thumb (Bell Krotoski, 2002). Indicate whether or not skin integrity has been compromised. Changes in sympathetic function should be documented like abnormal sweat patterns or skin blotching. Document any scars, calluses, wounds, and shiny or dry skin as these could all be indicators of sensory impairment. When sensation has been disrupted healing is decreased secondary to poor circulation.

Sensory assessments include specific tests for proprioception and stereognosis. Point localization can be assessed through tactile discrimination and the Semmes-Weinstein monofilament. Other assessments like threshold tests use sharp/dull items to assess protective sensation to identify deficits. Hyperalgesia can be identified using threshold tests. Temperature awareness is also assessed through protective sensory stimulus, if a deficit does exist in temperature recognition, then physical agent modalities (PAMS) will be contraindicated.

Functional test for sensory assessment includes the following:

- Static two-point discrimination (Novak, 2001)
- Moving two-point discrimination
- Localization of touch
- Localization of moving touch
- Moberg pickup test (Moberg, 1958)
- Nine Hole Peg Test

Sensory re-education occurs through desensitization which uses modified stimulation or PAMS that are tolerated by the client. The intervention will be performed in increments of 10 minutes at a frequency of up to four times per day. Protective sensation deficits increase the likelihood that injury will occur as a result of contact with cold or hot surfaces. Protective interventions to be taken by the occupational therapists are as follows:

- Protect the skin from exposure to sharp items and hot or cold items
- Decrease grip when holding objects
- Built-up handles (large handles)
- Limit activity time
- Assess skin integrity for possible compromises
- Moisturize skin frequently

Habituation occurs after multiple trials and repetition of stimuli that are not offensive to the client (Burleigh-Jacobs & Stehno-Bittel, 2002). Desensitization requires the use of graded stimuli that are tolerable to the client in small quantities (Skirven & Callahan, 2002).

Graded Tactile Discrimination starts with gross discrimination and ends with fine discrimination. The client will identify the stimulus using one of the three categories including:

- Same or different?
- How are they the same or different?
- Identify the item used

The assessment will begin with the client's eyes closed, then open, and repeat. The stimulus can be provided using varied methods like sandpaper, cotton, miscellaneous objects like screws or paperclips (Lundy-Ekman, 2007). Clients perform item retrieval from a shoebox filled with sand and small objects like coins or buttons (Lundy-Ekman, 2007). Other interventions for graded discrimination include Legos blocks or puzzles.

References

Bell Krotoski, J. A. (2002). Flexor tendon and peripheral nerve repair. *Journal of Hand Surgery, 7*, 83–109.

Burleigh-Jacobs, A., & Stehno-Bittel, L. (2002). Neuroplasticity. In L. Lundy-Ekman (Ed.) *Neuroscience: Fundamentals for rehabilitation* (2nd ed., pp. 67–80). Saunders.

Lundy-Ekman, L. (2007). *Neuroscience: Fundamentals for rehabilitation* (3rd ed.). Saunders.

Malaviya, G. N. (2003). Sensory perception in leprosy: Neurophysiological correlates (review). *International Journal of Leprosy and Other Mycobacterial Diseases, 71*, 119–124.

Moberg, E. (1958). Objective methods for determining the functional value of sensibility in the hand. *Journal of Bone & Joint Surgery, 40-B*, 454–476.

Novak, C. B. (2001). Evaluation of hand sensibility: A review. *Journal of Hand Therapy, 14*, 266–272.

Pedretti, L. W., Pendleton, H. M. H., & Schultz-Krohn, W. (2018). *Pedretti's occupational therapy: Practice skills for physical dysfunction* (8th ed.). Elsevier.

Skirven, T., & Callahan, A. D. (2002). Therapists' management of peripheral nerve injuries. In E. Mackin et al. (Eds.), *Rehabilitation of the hand and upper extremity* (5th ed., pp. 599–621). Mosby.

SECTION V
Orthopedic Conditions

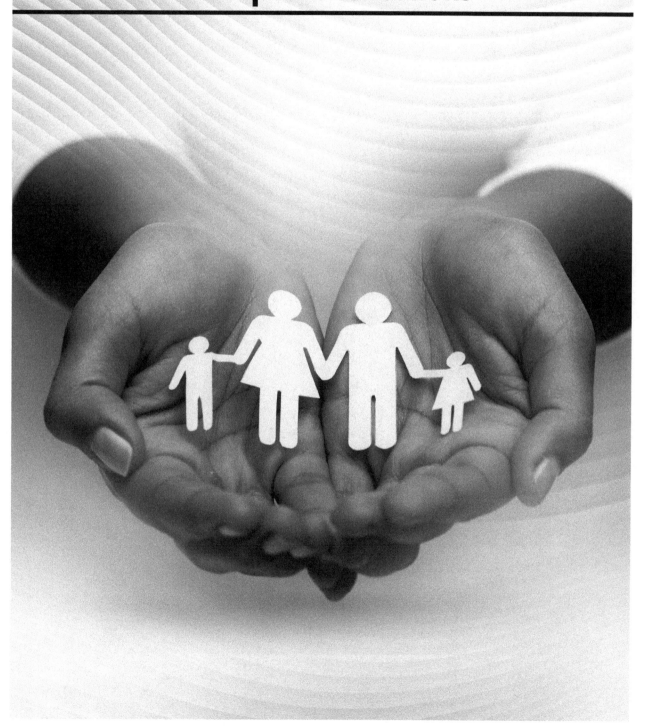

CHAPTER 10
Orthopedic Conditions for the Upper and Lower Extremities

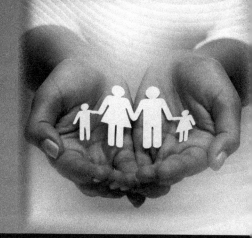

The upper extremity is complex with varied shoulder and elbow movements that allow the hand to be placed in several positions in space. Each joint in the upper extremity has a specific range of motion that allows it to move freely. The shoulder joint is a ball-and-socket joint with movement in three planes: It allows for

- flexion and extension in the sagittal plane
- lateral or horizontal abduction/adduction in the frontal plane
- internal and external rotation in the transverse plane

The clavicle and scapula are crucial in the rhythmic motion of the shoulder girdle. The shoulder is further complicated to treat and plan therapeutic interventions for because the joint is equally as unstable as it is movable, especially after an injury.

Acromioclavicular Joint

Because the shoulder allows for increased movement in the UE, in turn, proximal restriction of the shoulder will reduce distal freedom of movement in the upper extremity (Beim, 2000). When the sternoclavicular joint limits clavicular motion, it decreases the movement of the scapula, which limits functional use of the upper extremity (Beim, 2000). The sternoclavicular joint is a small freely movable synovial joint that attaches to the axial skeleton via bony attachments. The clavicle extends laterally and articulates with the lateral aspect of the spine of the scapula forming the **acromioclavicular joint (AC)**. Classic injury of the acromioclavicular joint is known as an AC split or shoulder separation. AC split injuries are common among athletes (Beim, 2000). The AC joint is not considered a true synovial joint because the joint capsule is non-existent. The capsule surrounds the joint and provides support to the joint that extends the length of the clavicle. Instead, the AC joint is supported via deltoid attachments both proximally and distally.

The shoulder girdle functions and moves with three degrees of freedom because of the interdependence of the sternum, clavicle, and scapula all of which work together to account for UE movement. The shoulder girdle also articulates with the thorax forming the scapulothoracic joint, which allows movement of the scapula in six directions including the following:

- Elevation and depression
- Protraction and retraction
- Upward and downward rotation

The range of motion of the shoulder depends heavily on the movement of the scapula. The body's ability to reach forward includes scapular protraction, elbow extension with shoulder flexion. Raising the hand overhead requires the ability to rotate the scapula upward, complete extension of the elbow, and shoulder flexion. Reaching behind the back also requires downward scapular rotation, internal rotation, and extension at the elbows.

51

SHOULDER ANATOMY

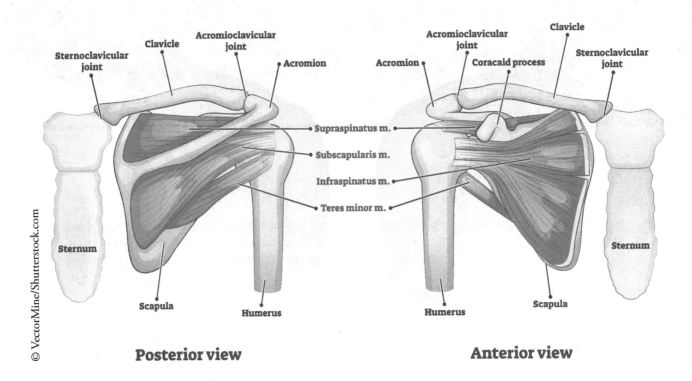

Glenoid Labrum and Ligaments

The glenoid labrum is made up of cartilage that increases the depth of the glenoid by 75% and 57% in the transverse plane (Cooper et al., 1992). The labrum is wedge-shaped and is modified with shoulder movement. The stability of the glenohumeral joint decreases by 20% if the labrum is absent (Yanogawa et al., 2008). The labrum also acts as a suction cup for the humeral head into the glenoid fossa to help reduce the risk of dislocation. The synovial sheath also adds to the support of the glenohumeral joints' stability as it inserts onto the anatomical neck of the humerus (Yanogawa et al., 2008). The glenohumeral joint is freely movable and the head of the humerus can be distracted from the glenoid fossa about a half-inch anteriorly and posteriorly. There are three folds of the joint capsule that make up the glenohumeral ligaments that stabilize the shoulder joint. They are as follows:

● Superior glenohumeral ligament—limits inferior dislocation of the humeral head
● Middle glenohumeral ligament—limits external rotation (missing in 30% of the population)
● Inferior glenohumeral ligament—stabilizes the joint capsule inferiorly and posteriorly

Scapulohumeral Rhythm

The shoulder girdle is further stabilized and strengthened by the muscles of the rotator cuff, capsular ligaments, coracohumeral ligament, glenoid labrum, and long head of the biceps. Keeping in mind that the shoulder girdle contributes its three degrees of motion partially to the range of motion available at the scapula, we must examine the shoulder girdle as a unit. Scapulohumeral rhythm is described as the complete range of motion of the shoulder considering both the glenohumeral joint and scapulothoracic joints (Crosbie et al., 2008). The combined range of motion of the shoulder is 180 degrees versus the 120 degrees of motion with the scapulothoracic joint. The rhythm between the glenohumeral joint and scapulothoracic joint is 2:1 (Crosbie et al., 2008), which means for every 2 degrees of shoulder flexion or abduction, the scapula must rotate upward approximately 1 degree (Crosbie et al., 2008). This ratio applies to shoulder extension as well.

Shoulder Joint

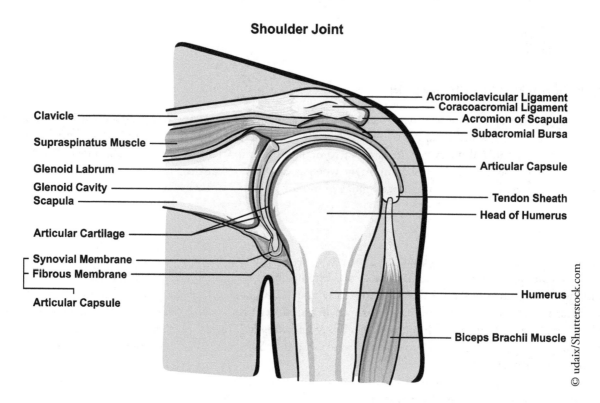

Clavicle

Supraspinatus Muscle

Glenoid Labrum

Glenoid Cavity

Scapula

Articular Cartilage

Synovial Membrane

Fibrous Membrane

Articular Capsule

Acromioclavicular Ligament

Coracoacromial Ligament

Acromion of Scapula

Subacromial Bursa

Articular Capsule

Tendon Sheath

Head of Humerus

Humerus

Biceps Brachii Muscle

© udaix/Shutterstock.com

While assessing shoulder movement, it is imperative to ensure that the client has enough external rotation in the joint before assessing flexion and upward rotation of the scapula. Any alterations in the motion of the scapula can be related to declines in serratus anterior muscle activity, increases in upper trapezius muscle activity, or unbalanced force between the upper and lower trapezius muscles. It is important to ensure appropriate muscle balance to demonstrate strength and flexibility.

The muscles that assist in the movement of the shoulder:

- Levator scapulae—scapular elevation
- Rhomboid—retracts the scapula and rotates to depress the glenoid fossa.
- Trapezius—rotation, retraction, elevation, and depression of the scapula

Rotator Cuff

The muscles of the rotator cuff support the humeral head in the glenoid fossa (Terry & Chopp, 2000). The muscles of the rotator cuff include the following:

- Supraspinatus
- Infraspinatus
- Teres minor
- Subscapularis

The large medial rotators of the humerus are the following:

- Subscapularis
- Latissimus Dorsi

Rotator Cuff Muscles

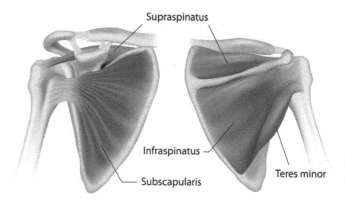

Supraspinatus

Infraspinatus

Subscapularis

Teres minor

Anterior view

Posterior view

© Alila Medical Media/Shutterstock.com

- Teres Major
- Pectoralis Major

Upward Rotation of the Scapula

The fibers of the trapezius muscles help to stabilize the scapula, the serratus anterior protracts the inferior/anterior border of the scapula, while the upper trapezius fibers elevate the lateral angle of the scapula. Therefore, the upward rotation of the scapula also elevates the lateral acromion and is important to prevent the impingement from the lateral border of the scapula. It is also important when assessing ROM at the shoulder to ensure that the client is not compensating for a poor glenohumeral range of motion.

Shoulder Pain

Hemiplegic shoulder pain complaints account for about 21 million doctor's visits in the United States. One of the most common pain syndromes is subacromial impingement syndrome, which is best described as the tendon rubbing underneath the shoulder blade (Cowderoy et al., 2009). This rubbing produces muscle instability and weakness in the lower and middle trapezius muscle group, serratus anterior, infraspinatus, and deltoid muscles (Cowderoy et al., 2009). In addition to the rubbing and muscle imbalance, there is also increased muscle tone in the upper trapezius, pectoralis group, and levator scapulae. Subacromial impingement occurs more often with people who have neglect due to a stroke.

Decreased sensation and increased pain affect the shoulder girdle's movement, which also makes it difficult to specify the exact cause of pain. Common pain types include the following:

- Neuromuscular pain—dull ache
- Glenohumeral impingement—sharp radiating pain
- Neuropathic pain—constant burning sensation

Shoulder pain occurs frequently with clients who have spasticity and flaccidity (Shah et al., 2008; Zeferino & Aycock, 2010). Evidence shows that the highest correlation for the development of shoulder pain occurs in people who have used an overhead pulley (Kumar et al., 1990). Decreased external rotation at the shoulder has also been associated with pain.

Causes for Shoulder Pain

Anatomical Site	Mechanism
Muscle	Muscle imbalance Impingement (rotator cuff) Contractures Subscapularis and Pectoralis spasticity
Joint	Subluxation (weak correlation)
Bursa/tendon	Bursitis/Tendonitis
Joint capsule	Frozen or contracted shoulder (adhesive capsulitis)
Other	Shoulder-hand syndrome (complex regional pain syndrome (CRPS)

Soft Tissue Injuries

Soft tissue injuries can be caused by several different reasons primarily because the shoulder is fundamentally unstable and is a freely movable joint. Pain can be caused by the gravity and weight of the arm pulling down on the humeral head thereby displacing it from the glenoid fossa. Another cause for shoulder pain is poor handling by caregivers or poor positioning of the arm. Positioning needs should be addressed to help prevent subluxation using orthosis. Other causes can include pinching of the tissue due to lapse in technique or decreased range of motion (Kumar et al., 1990).

Other deficits occur in the upper extremity due to soft tissue damage such as contractures and deformities. Weakness and sensation impairments can also lead to upper extremity dysfunction or pain. Some people have experienced soft tissue damage in the shoulder secondary to poor quality of movement, absence of voluntary motor control, and loss of biomechanical alignment.

Assessment

The initial step in the assessment phase for occupational therapy is to observe the client's posture, arm placement, and upper extremity movement. Inquire with the client about pain levels and location. This is an important detail when developing a treatment intervention for shoulder dysfunction. Assess for subluxation and scapula position before you begin any range of motion. After subluxation assessment, the OT should evaluate a passive range of motion, starting with external rotation then moving through the remaining ranges at the shoulder. Complete a manual muscle test for the rotator cuff muscles and other supporting musculature of the shoulder girdle through isolated movements. Sensation assessment, awareness/neglect, and other outcome measures can be completed in the final stages of the evaluation. The hierarchy can be modified as needed according to the specific needs of the client for much of the shoulder assessment, excluding the range of motion assessment.

Postural Alignment

Clients present with postural changes secondary to CVA, orthopedic changes, and many other degenerative types of disease processes. These clients can present clinically with deficits in the following:

- trunk control, midline orientation
- midline orientation
- cognitive deficits
- visual deficits
- left inattention

Trunk malalignment can also be due to weak cervical flexors, weak rhomboids, and weak lower traps. The natural alignment of the trunk is very important for the initiation of the muscles that move the humerus and scapula. During the evaluation of the shoulder, it is very important to have the client maintain correct alignment throughout the assessment process. A second cause for trunk malalignment is tight occipital muscles, upper trapezius, levator scapulae, and pectoralis muscles will produce postural deficits.

Subluxation

According to Pedretti, subluxation is best described as a palpable gap between the acromion and humeral head. This gap is caused by the mechanical forces applied to the shoulder, therefore affecting the integrity of the glenohumeral joint. In the beginning stages of shoulder subluxation, the client experiences little pain, but as the gap grows larger between the acromion and the humeral head, the stress force applied to the joint increases the pain response. Most clients present with subluxation due to loss of joint capsule integrity secondary to poor upper extremity positioning following a CVA.

Compression stresses occur with abduction and flexion of a subluxed shoulder in the absence of sufficient scapulohumeral rhythm. The stability of a subluxed shoulder is achieved by the fibro tendinous sleeve of the rotator cuff which will maintain the humeral head in the glenoid cavity. Collectively, the joint capsule, supraspinatus, and posterior deltoid muscles work together to prevent subluxation. Occupational therapists can stimulate the posterior deltoid and supraspinatus to aid in reducing subluxation. Other methods of prevention of subluxation

SHOULDER SUBLUXATION

NORMAL POSITION OF THE SHOULDER

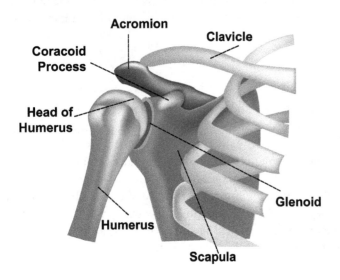

SHOULDER SUBLUXATION

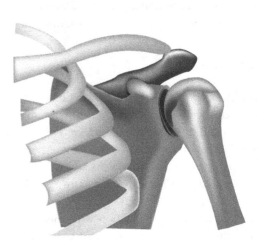

© La vector/Shutterstock.com

include optimal scapular position achieved by strengthening the upward rotators of the scapula. The most common intervention for subluxation prevention is to use an orthosis or sling to support the upper extremity. When the joint capsule is absent the surrounding muscle is unable to recover from eccentric contraction. The periarticular tissue is overstretched due to the increase in pain receptors in the ligaments and capsule. The overstretching can also result in painful ischemia in the tendons.

There are three types of subluxation:

- **Inferior**—Downward rotation of the scapula with abduction and medial rotation of the humeral head below the inferior lip of fossa.
- **Anterior**—Downward rotation and elevation of the scapula, hyperextension and medial rotation of the humeral head inferior and forward relative to the glenoid fossa.
- **Superior**—Elevation and abduction of the scapula, medial rotation and abduction of the humerus, and humeral head wedged under the coracoid process of the scapula. Also, the result of increased deltoid activity without the activation of the rotator cuff to hold the humeral head down during flexion.

In order to measure the size of a subluxation, you must measure the space between the acromion process of the scapula and the head of the humerus. A rule of thumb: *always* compare the unaffected side to the affected side to establish a baseline. Palpate around the shoulder joint using the fingers and use centimeters as the unit of measurement.

Scapular Winging

According to Pedretti, scapular winging can be caused by injury to the long thoracic nerve or weakness of the serratus anterior muscle which results in medial winging of the scapula. Other causes for scapular winging are weakness in the trapezius and rhomboid muscles. If the medial border of the scapula is not stable, then the pectoralis minor pulls on the coracoid process of the scapula during inhalation. Other contributing factors of medial border scapular winging include denervation or paralysis of the thoracic wall muscles that protract resulting in the scapula lifting from the thoracic wall.

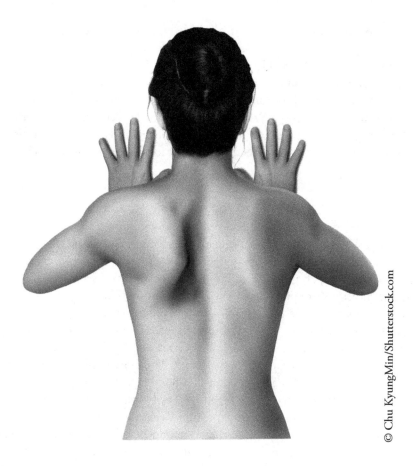

Assessment of the scapula

Scapular alignment is crucial when assessing the scapula. Palpate the spine of the scapula, inferior angle, and position of the medial border of the scapula. Active scapula movement will depend heavily on the proper alignment. Also assess all ranges of motion for the scapula including elevation/depression and protraction/retraction. **Scaption** is the combined movement of elevation and either internal rotation or external rotation of the scapula. The scapula's plane of movement is 30–45 degrees anterior to the frontal plane. Through scaption, clients can achieve length-tension in the anterior and posterior muscle capsules that improves stability. Scaption in conjunction with the upper extremities in anatomical position decreases the risk of shoulder impingement during shoulder abduction. The scapula's anatomical position is described as having the following:

- vertebral border parallel to the spine
- two to three fingers from the midline of the thorax
- between the 2nd and 7th thoracic vertebrae
- 30 degrees anterior to the frontal plane with a 10-degree anterior tilt

Common malalignments of the scapula can present as downward rotation with winging of the medial border. Glenohumeral joint dysfunction with lateral flexion of the trunk and downward rotation of the scapula results in depression and subluxation. Other scapula dysfunction presents as upper extremity flexion synergy pattern with internal rotation and adduction with elbow flexion, forearm pronation, wrist flexion and ulnar deviation and finger flexion.

Lower Extremity Injury

The hip and knee are both described as large weight-bearing joints. When these types of joints are unstable for an extended period, participation in the purposeful activity is diminished. The group is at highest risk for hip fractures secondary to decreased mobility and osteoporosis in the elderly. Decreased flexibility, decline in strength, slower reaction times, and assistive devices impair the elderly population's mobility. Research has shown that women are at higher risk for hip fracture than men. Most elderly people are fearful of falling and therefore they are more cautious when ambulating. Other significant reasons for increased falls in the elderly are the inappropriate use of assistive devices and low vision. Lower extremity injuries and joint replacements are common in those who present with rheumatic diseases and osteoarthritis. OT's role in the rehabilitation process for clients who suffer lower extremity injuries is improving safety, increasing independence, and completion of purposeful tasks. OTs can also provide community-based resources for the elderly to assist in fall reduction (Centers for Disease Control and Prevention, n.d.).

Medical Management

Fractures happen because the bone can no longer absorb tension, compression, or shearing forces have been exhausted (Delisa & Gans, 2010). Cells that mend broken bones are called osteoblasts. Osteoblasts and good blood supply both promote healing. Healthy blood supply is essential to provide surrounding cells with adequate oxygen to enhance healing. Following surgery, the repaired bone is protected by pins and wires. In some cases, it is necessary to provide an abductor orthosis to protect the hip or a knee immobilizer to protect the knee.

The goal of fracture management is to decrease pain, obtain an optimal bone position, healing, and renew independent function. Fracture reduction involves restoring the bone fragments to normal alignment, by a closed (manipulation) or an open (surgical) procedure (Delisa & Gans, 2010). The closed reduction procedure is completed by a doctor who applies force to the misaligned bone. The closed reduction procedure is maintained by using braces, cast, traction, or fixators. Open reduction of a fracture site is completed via surgery to improve the alignment of bone pieces. The pieces of bone are held together by pins, rods, screws, nails, and plates. Weight-bearing precautions are always indicated after each procedure (Delisa & Gans, 2010).

Weight-bearing restrictions vary depending on the severity, type of injury, and location of the damage. Clients who have surgical procedures or manipulative procedures both must follow weight-bearing precautions. The lowest level of weight-bearing is non-weight-bearing (NWB), which implies absolutely no weight on the involved extremity. The next level is toe-touch weight-bearing (TTWB) or touchdown weight-bearing, which implies only the toe can be placed down to support the client when standing and 90% of the client's weight is placed on the unaffected extremity. The next restriction is partial weight-bearing (PWB), which implies only 50% of weight can be placed on the affected extremity. Weight-bearing as tolerated (WBAT) implies that it is up to the client to decide how much weight will be placed on the affected extremity. The final restriction is full weight-bearing (FWB), which implies that 100% of the client's weight can be placed on the affected extremity. Weight-bearing restrictions are decreased as the reduction site heals (Canale & Beaty, 2007).

Etiology

The most common cause of fractures is trauma, usually secondary to a fall. Occupational therapists should observe the client's environment for potential falls such as lighting hazards, throw rugs, and unmarked steps. Other environmental hazards include excessive clutter, extension cords, and small pets. Osteoporosis is described as a bone disease that is marked with decreased bone density and is common in the vertebral bodies, the neck of the femur, the humerus, and the distal end of the radius. Osteoporosis affects mostly older adults. With osteoporosis the bone is very thin and porous making it fragile and more prone to fractures secondary to a traumatic fall. Pathologic fractures happen when the bone is weak due to disease or tumor, such as osteomyelitis or malignant neoplasms (Delisa & Gans, 2010).

There are three types of hip fractures:

- Femoral neck fractures
- Intertrochanteric fractures
- Subtrochanteric fractures

Femoral neck fractures can occur in several different locations. There is a sub-capital fracture, a transcervical fracture, and a basilar fracture. These fractures happen more often with women than with men secondary to

FEMORAL NECK FRACTURE

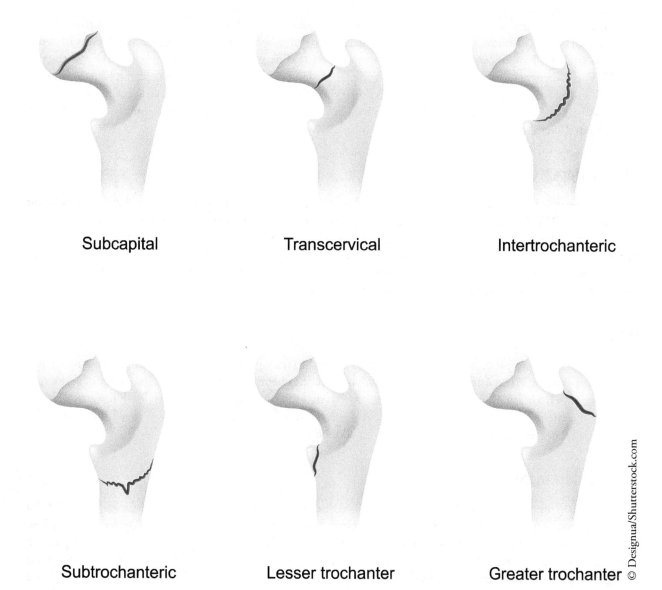

Subcapital   Transcervical   Intertrochanteric

Subtrochanteric   Lesser trochanter   Greater trochanter © Designua/Shutterstock.com

osteoporosis. Femoral neck fractures can also be due to rotation or trauma which makes them more difficult to treat if the blood supply is insufficient, low bone density, and deteriorating periosteum covering the bone (Larson et al., 1996). When the blood supply is intact, and the fracture is moderate to minimal the physician uses pinning (screw and plate). When the femoral neck is severely displaced or has decreased blood supply (avascular necrosis), or slow healing fracture, and degenerative joint disease the femoral head is surgically removed and replaced with an endoprosthesis called a hemiarthroplasty (Melvin & Gall, 1999; Richardson & Iglarsh, 1994). There is a vast selection of endoprosthesis choices each with pros and cons. The posterolateral approach procedure begins at the posterior aspect of the hip and then around the lateral surface of the hip. The anterolateral approach is performed starting on the anterior aspect of the hip and then around the lateral surface. Post-surgical movement of the affected extremity begins as early as 1 day after surgery (Melvin & Gall, 1999; Richardson & Iglarsh, 1994; Singh et al., 2010).

An intertrochanteric fracture occurs between the greater and lesser trochanter and is extracapsular which means outside the articular capsule of the hip joint. Like many fractures, an intertrochanteric fracture has a higher occurrence in women than in men. Intertrochanteric fractures often occur secondary to direct force to the trochanter. To repair an intertrochanteric fracture physician will perform an ORIF via a nail or a compression screw. The weight-bearing restrictions should be maintained up to 4 months post operation during ambulation and transfers (Canale & Beaty, 2007). Clients are out of bed as early as 1-day post-operation.

Subtrochanteric fractures occur 1 to 2 inches below the lesser trochanter, due to direct force trauma such as a fall, MVA, or sports. Subtrochanteric fractures usually occur in people who are younger than 60 years of age or elderly people who have a low impact fall (Nieves et al., 2010). The most common treatment is skeletal traction and ORIF replacement. A nail or intramedullary rod placed along the lateral aspect of the hip can be used to repair the break in the bone (Delisa & Gans, 2010). Occupational therapists should note additional conditions such as edema, soft tissue injury, or bruising can occur, which can cause pain or discomfort at the surgical site (Delisa & Gans, 2010; Richardson & Iglarsh, 1994).

Joint Replacement

Chronic degenerative diseases will cause damage and often require surgery such as rheumatoid arthritis (RA) and osteoarthritis (OA). Degenerative changes can also be caused by congenital defects, trauma, or any disease that cause injury to the articular cartilage. Normally, large weight-bearing joints are affected by degenerative diseases, such as the hip, knee, and lumbar spine. There are several other diseases such as lupus, cancer, and RA that can have an effect on these large weight-bearing joints usually due to medications used to treat the diseases. The medications can affect the blood supply to the bone cells causing avascular necrosis (AVN; Opitz, 1990).

Hip Replacement

There are two common procedure approaches used to repair hip fractures: the anterolateral approach and the posterolateral approach. When using the anterolateral approach, the client is unsteady in external rotation, adduction, and extension. Hip precautions include no adduction, external rotation, and no extension. With the posterolateral approach the client has weakness in hip flexion. Hip precautions for the posterolateral approach include no hip flexion past 90 degrees, no internal rotation, and no adduction.

Knee Replacement

There are two common types of knee replacement surgeries performed in the United States each year. The first is the total knee arthroplasty (TKA) which is performed because osteoarthritis, some type of degenerative joint disease, or trauma is present in two or more compartments of the knee. TKA is performed to decrease pain, increase range of motion in the knee, and ensure alignment and support the joint. During the TKA, the injured or damaged bone is cut away and a prosthesis is attached. The second procedure is called a unicompartmental knee arthroplasty, which is necessary if damage exists medially or laterally in compartments between the femur and tibia.

OT Role

The role of occupational therapy in lower extremity joint replacement always begins with an explanation of who you are, what your expectations are for the client. Be sure to provide clear instructions that the client understands. Complete an occupational profile and establish a baseline for function. Observe the client performing ADLs and basic skills to justify goals and interventions. Educating the family and caregiver should always be incorporated into the plan of care for these clients.

Interventions

Interventions for lower extremity injuries post-surgically include bed mobility and the use of adaptive equipment for positioning in the bed. An abductor wedge is most used to maintain proper joint alignment. Other adaptive equipment includes bedside commodes (BSC) to improve safety during toileting. Make sure that the BSC is high enough to accommodate the pressure at the hip when seated. Non-skid surfaces and grab bars can also be installed in the shower to decrease fall risk following lower extremity surgery. Patients should only shower in a standing position or using a shower chair/bench, no baths, as it would not comply with hip precautions. When transferring use flat surfaces to avoid unnecessary weight shifting, which causes discomfort. ADLs are always an ongoing component of the rehabilitation process and must be assessed throughout the duration of therapeutic intervention.

Special Equipment

Lower extremity surgeries require the use of many types of special equipment. A hemovac is a plastic drain that is inserted into the surgical site. An abduction wedge is a triangular-shaped, foam pillow that is inserted between the thighs to maintain optimal hip position following a THA. Balance suspension is a pulley system used to distribute weight evenly; it is like traction. Reclining wheelchairs have adjustable backs for increased comfort following a lower extremity surgery. Sequential compression devices (SCD) are inflatable garments applied to the legs to reduce the risk for blood clots after surgery. Anti-embolus hose (TED) are thick hose-like garments made to minimize the risk for blood clots after surgery. Client-controlled IV is an epidural line that is controlled by the client by pushing a button to deliver a pre-set amount of medication.

References

Beim, G. M. (2000). Acromioclavicular joint injuries. *Journal of Athletic Training, 35*(3), 261–267.

Canale, S. T., & Beaty, J. H. (2007). *Campbell's operative orthopedics* (11th ed.). Mosby.

Centers for Disease Control and Prevention. (n.d.). *STEADI: Older adult fall prevention.* http://www.cdc.gov/steadi/index.html

Cooper, D. E., Arnoczky, S. P., O'Brien, S. J., Warren, R. F., DiCarlo, E., & Allen, A. A. (1992). Anatomy, histology, and vascularity of the glenoid labrum. An anatomical study. *Journal of Bone and Joint Surgery, 74*(1), 46–52.

Cowderoy, G. A., Lisle, D. A., & O'Connell, P. T. (2009). Overuse and impingement syndromes of the shoulder in the athlete. *Magnetic Resonance Imaging Clinics of North America, 17*(4), 577–593. doi:10.1016/j.mric.2009.06.003

Crosbie, J., Kilbreath, S. L., Hollmann, L., & York, S. (2008). Scapulohumeral rhythm and associated spinal motion. *Clinical Biomechanics, 23*(2), 184–192.

Delisa, J., & Gans, B. (2010). *Rehabilitation medicine: Principles and practice* (5th ed.). JB Lippincott.

Kumar, R., Metter, E. J., Mehta, A. J., & Chew, T. (1990). Shoulder pain in hemiplegia. The role of exercise. *American Journal of Physical Medicine & Rehabilitation, 69*(4), 205–208. doi:10.1097/00002060-199008000-00007

Larson, K. O., Stevens-Ratchford, R., Pedretti, L., & Crabtree, J. (Eds.) (1996). *Role of occupational therapy with the elderly.* American Occupational Therapy Association.

Melvin, J., & Gall, V. (1999). *Rheumatic rehabilitation series: Surgical rehabilitation* (vol 5). American Occupational Therapy Association.

Nieves, J. W., Bilezikian, J. P., Lane, J. M., Einhorn, T. A., Wang, Y., Steinbuch, M., & Cosman, F. (2010). Fragility fractures of the hip and femur: Incidence and patient characteristics. *Osteoporosis International, 21*, 399–408.

Opitz, J. (1990). Reconstructive surgery of the extremities. In F. Kottle & J. Lehmann (Eds.) *Krusen's handbook of physical medicine and rehabilitation* (4th ed.). WB Saunders.

Richardson, J. K., & Iglarsh, Z. A. (1994). *Clinical orthopaedic physical therapy.* WB Saunders.

Shah, R. R., Haghpanah, S., Elovic, E. P., Flanagan, S. R., Behnegar, A., Nguyen, V., Page, S. J., Fang, Z.-P., & Chae, J. (2008). MRI findings in the painful poststroke shoulder. *Stroke, 39*(6), 1808–1813. https://doi.org/10.1161/STROKEAHA.107.502187

Singh, J., Sloan, J., & Johanson, N. (2010). Challenges with health-related quality of life assessment in arthroplasty patients: problems and solutions. *Journal of the American Academy of Orthopaedic Surgeons, 18*, 72–82.

Terry, G. C., & Chopp, T. M. (2000). Functional anatomy of the shoulder. *Journal of Athletic Training, 35*(3), 248–255.

Yanagawa, T., Goodwin, C. J., Shelburne, K. B., Giphart, J. E., Torry, M. R., & Pandy, M. G. (2008). Contributions of the individual muscles of the shoulder to glenohumeral joint stability during abduction. *Journal of Biomechanical Engineering, 130*(2), 021024. https://doi.org/10.1115/1.2903422

Zeferino, S. I., & Aycock, D. M. (2010). Poststroke shoulder pain: Inevitable or preventable? *Rehabilitation Nursing Journal, 35*(4), 147–151. doi:10.1002/j.2048-7940.2010.tb00040.x

CHAPTER 11
Orthotics and Prosthetics

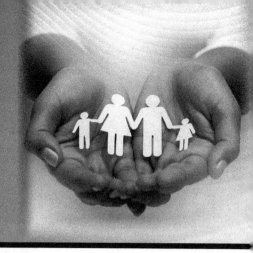

Pedretti states that an orthosis is a force system designed to control, correct, or compensate for a bone deformity (Anderson et al., 1994). There are several indications for splinting a joint or a body part. A splint is an orthopedic device used for immobilization, restraining, or supporting a joint or a body part. Orthosis is the term used by healthcare professionals during clinical practice for devices such as splints or casts (Anderson et al., 1994). An orthotist makes suspension arm devices and occupational therapists modify the devices and educate the clients on how to use them. Splints are designed to improve occupational performances (AOTA, 2014).

According to https://medical-dictionary.thefreedictionary.com/prosthetics, prosthetics involve the use of artificial limbs to increase the function and way of life for people who have lost limbs. The prosthesis is a one-of-a-kind combination of special materials and unique designs to facilitate the functional needs of the client. The prosthetic device is designed to address the functional deficits of each client. For example, the devices are designed to improve ADL performance and to complete gardening. The artificial limb outlines occupational exercises that include reaching and grasping. Splints and prosthetics both can improve the functional independence of those people who need them.

Amputations are the result of diseases, injuries, infections, and congenital defects. The surgical removal of an extremity secondary to injury or disease is referred to as an acquired amputation. Robert King is a Desert Storm and Iraqi war veteran. He lost his upper left forearm caused by an improvised explosive device (IED) roadside bomb. An IED causes loss of limbs as well as loss of life. They also cause traumatic brain injuries, post-traumatic stress disorder, and blast injury. A blast injury can cause loss of hearing, tinnitus, and vertigo. Military veterans that have lost limbs in combat and training are given the opportunity to obtain artificial limbs. Instead of the traditional and pirate-style hooks, today's amputees get the choice of robot-like arms. These new devices may look like the real thing—but they still can't act like real arms. Veterans attend rehabilitation training to learn how to insert the limb into their life. Especially if they use kitchen utensils in a lab to teach them how to perform operations to eat, cook, and clean. Also, the veteran learns how to grasp objects such as bottles, drinking glasses, and plates (King, Personal Conversation, March 23, 2021).

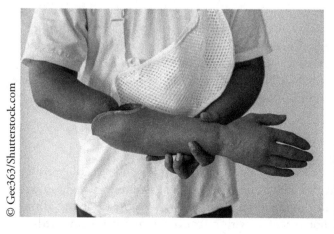

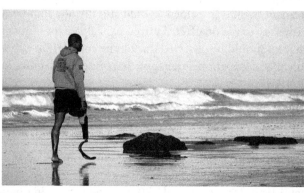

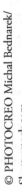

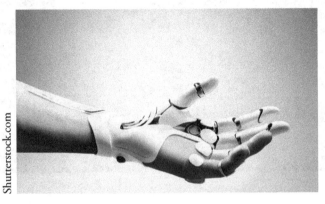

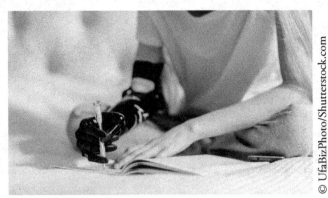

Hand splints

The hand function is one of the most important parts of the human body's function. We use our hands more often than we use any other body parts. Learning to use the hands begins very early in life and continues throughout development. This learned use of the hands occurs via the relationship to the brain, which is a complicated nervous system and synaptic connections. The hand and shoulder function together to obtain balance and organized movements. The elbow and wrist must both work together to maintain the hand's position in space. Any brain abnormalities can lead to deficits in hand movement. Hand abnormalities affect the complete person mentally, physically, and emotionally. Splints are one of the most essential devices that occupational therapists use to decrease or remedy abnormalities or to renew or modify functions.

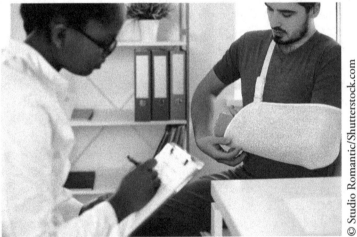

OT Role

Occupational therapists should begin by completing an activity analysis to identify deficits in occupational performances. The assessment should also include standardized tests and outcomes, and a comparison of the affected extremity to the unaffected extremity. Palpate for bony prominences and anatomical structures. The client's biomechanics should be observed during the completion of ADL and IADL tasks. The fabrication of splints is a unique role that occupational therapists have in the rehabilitation process (Hollister & Giurintano, 1999).

Anatomy of the hand

The hand and wrist collectively are made up of 27 bones and they all aid in the movement and versatility of the arm and hand. The wrist is intricate and is made up of the distal ulna and radius and the two rows of eight carpal bones. These carpal bones create a concave transverse arch, and the distal radius assists with the flexibility of the hand (van der Heide et al., 2014). The distal ulna does not articulate with carpal bones and it is connected to the wrist by way of the collateral ligament, which assists in supporting the wrist and restricts radial deviation. The wrist also permits the largest arc of motion than any other joints besides the ankle.

Upper extremity movement is further complicated due to wrist extension allowing for radial deviation and supination. Ulnar deviation and pronation are necessary to perform wrist flexion. The anatomy of the wrist is complex. The distal row of carpal bones is composed of the trapezium, trapezoid, capitate, and hamate, while the proximal row is made up of the scaphoid, lunate, and triquetrum. Motion at the wrist is like a "floating" motion and happens during all stages of movement. It is limited only by the carpal ligaments. Wrist tenodesis is a movement phenomenon in which the opposite motion of the wrist and fingers that occurs during the active or passive wrist flexion and extension. Wrist extension produces finger flexion, and wrist flexion producing finger extension.

MP and MCP Joints

The metacarpal bones articulate with the carpal bones proximally and with the phalanges distally. Because the wrist forms a cone shape when it closes, the ulnar 2 digits of the hand meet the palm first when making a fist, then the radial digits follow. This phenomenon is important when creating the distal trim lines for splints when the goal is full MP flexion. Be sure that the trim lines along the ulnar border are not too long as it will limit flexion of the 4th and 5th digits. If the trim lines are too long, they can limit the client's ability to grasp large objects and movement will be limited. When the trim lines are of appropriate length movement is not restricted and full MP flexion is attainable. Forearm rotation includes supination and pronation. These are essential for wrist splint fabrication. Splints are usually worn on the forearm in pronation but are simple to create in supination.

Ligamental structures of the hand and wrist

Ligaments of the hand and wrist perform as checkreins, because they limit the motion at the wrist. The ligaments of the hand and wrist are the palmar, radial, and ulnar. The support and flexibility of the thumb are based on the

Muscles of the Forearm
(right arm, posterior compartment)

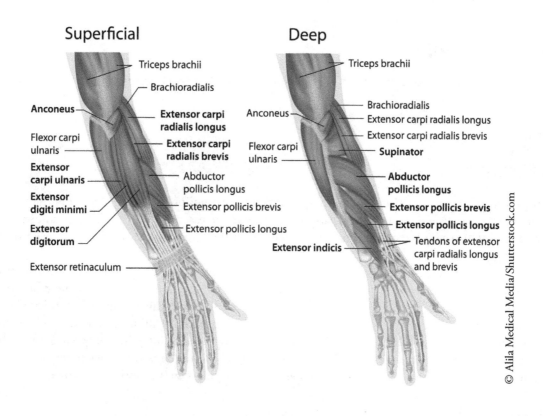

© Alila Medical Media/Shutterstock.com

quality of these ligaments. Both the radial and ulnar collateral ligaments sustain dorsal balance. Interruption of any of these ligaments will cause pain, reduce strength, and limit function.

Prehension and Grasp

Prehension is the capacity to apply sufficient force from the hand to grasp an object. Grasp is described as a hand position that enables the palm to contact the surface of objects by flexing the digits. Some splints are used to increase prehension. Lateral prehension is described as pad of thumb is in direct contact with the radial side of the middle or distal finger. A common daily use for lateral prehension is holding chopsticks or turning a key. Palmar prehension is described as the thumb placed in opposition to the index and long fingers. This pattern is also called as the "three-jaw chuck" and is used to pick up items from a flat surface. Tip prehension presents as the IP joint of the thumb and DIP and PIP joints of the finger are flexed to promote tip-to-tip prehension (Pedretti et al., 2018).

Hand Splinting

Splint application directly affects the transmission of the force of motion. A balanced line that is motionless when the bones of a joint move in relationship to one another is called the axis of motion (Hollister & Giurintano, 1999). When splints have a single axis, joint motion happens in one plane. The PIP is a single-axis joint. In multi-axis joints the motion occurs in multiple planes at once. Splints with a movable hinge or coil have a single axle. Proper alignment of the hinge of the joint with single-axis splints is crucial to achieve a full range of motion.

Force

According to Pedretti, force is the effects that materials and their dynamic components have on bone and tissue. Force is the measurement of stress, friction, and torque. Stress is the opposition to any force that impairs or changes tissue. Shear stress is created when force is applied in opposing directions. Friction is created when one surface prohibits the gliding of a surface on another. Torque is a measure of the force that results in the rotation of a lever around an axis. Translational forces are created when the angle of the lever arm's approach is less than 90 degrees or greater than 90 degrees.

Splint Types by Function

There are many types of hand splints use in rehabilitation. Some of the common types are the following:

- static
- serial static
- dynamic
- static progressive

Dynamic splints are composed of multiple strong parts that create motion. Static splints do not move and restrict a joint or a body part. A serial splint creates a slow progressive increase in ROM by frequent adjustments of the splint or cast. A static splint is composed of a static component that modifies the amount or angle of traction acting on a part.

Splints are also created for specific reasons, for example some splints are organized according to articular or non-articular. Some splints are put into three categories such as restriction, immobilization, and mobilization. Restriction splints decrease ROM and do not limit joint motion. A PIP block is an example of a restriction splint. Immobilization splints limit motion completely and can be ordered to minimize injury, rest, to decrease inflammation or pain, and positioning to promote healing after surgery. A resting hand splint is an example of an immobilization splint. Mobilization splints are designed to improve limited ROM or to renew or change functions. These splints have been fabricated to assist a frail muscle or compensate for motion loss (Pedretti et al., 2018).

Adhering to splinting protocols is essential. Obedience and intrinsic motivation are crucial elements to achieving established outcomes for splinting. When educating a client about donning and doffing a splint, be sure that the client understands exactly what should be done. If the client has a caregiver education of the caregiver is also essential. Completing a skin assessment is important for splinting as hypersensitivity may prevent a client from tolerating a specific splint. Ensure that the client and caregivers are informed about the wear schedule for all splints (Pedretti et al., 2018).

Splint Making Process

The first step is to create a pattern by tracing the outline of the client's hand while it lies on a flat surface. The second step is to choose material appropriate for the type of splint you want to fabricate. Splint material comes in multiple forms and the characteristics vary according to the type. Resistance to stretch is how a material opposes pulling or stretching. This characteristic increases the level of control the OT will have over the material. Conformability or drape is described as how easily a material stretches. Splint materials with this characteristic form a tighter bond to the client's extremity than other materials. Memory is the ability of a material when it is heated to return to the original form or shape after being sculpted. Rigidity is present when the material is cold and force is applied, it could crack. If the material is cold, when force is applied then it bends without cracking. Bonding is the ability to adhere to itself when the material has been warmed and joined together. Self-sealing edges are round and seal themselves when warmed material is cut. Soft splint materials provide partial motion around a joint, yet still limit or protect the part. Step three is to identify the kind of traction that will move or stabilize the joint(s). The traction component can be dynamic, elastic, hinge, or static. Dynamic traction mobilizes a joint via a resistant force connected to an outrigger or a coil. Static traction limits motion at the joint. When splints are fabricated for immobilization, they are protecting, resting, or positioning a body part. Continuous adjustments of the end joint range of splints are called static serial traction. This type of splint uses a gradual approach for improving the range of motion (Pedretti et al., 2018).

Splint Types by material

Forearm-based and hand-based splints are made from material with a high level of conformability. Forearm-based splints are used to remold scar tissue, restrict or promote healing in tissue with an acute disease process, and to construct the base of a dynamic splint. Large upper and lower extremity splints are constructed with high resilience materials for improved stability to handle large parts. Large upper and lower extremity splints are used to construct splints for the knee, shoulder, ankle, or elbow. Palpate for bony prominences and add cushion splint to balance pressure. Circumferential splints are devised to wrap completely around the body part. These splints are made from materials with high levels of memory, which allows them to stretch without thinning. A static progressive traction splint has a mechanism within the splint to modify the amount of traction, like Velcro or buckles. Occupational therapists should apply enough force to produce motion. Make sure you do not overexert force on a joint as this extra force could cause low blood oxygen levels. OTS must always use their best clinical judgment when working with splints. The amount of force is dependent on the length of time the contracture has been present, the severity of muscle tone, demographics about the client, and the location of the contracture. The creep of splint material is best described as the stress applied to tissue over an extended period and relaxed. The goal is that the tissue will adjust to the new shape instead of assuming the original shape. The elastic limit of tissue is the point at which tissue stretch will cause pain and injury can occur. Tissue growth is described as when living cells detect stress and elastin fibers are active and gradually absorb and distribute with altered bonding patterns with no creep or inflammation. Step four is to identify a splint design with a specific feature designed for the client. One unique technique used to prepare a joint for splinting is stress relaxation, which is when the muscle is stretched to its max limit and the position is sustained for brief periods of time. Scar tissue remodeling is an example of splint fabrication for a specific need of the client. Scar tissue has adherent tendencies by attaching to the connective tissue surrounding an injury or at the surgical site, and then restricting the movement of a specific area. Physical agent modalities with a heat component can improve tissue response and flexibility, thereby improving a muscles' ability to elongate. The resting hand splint positions the hand in a functional hand position. The objective of this splint is to maintain the soft tissue in the middle range to achieve ideal mobility and limit the shortening of the soft tissue (Pedretti et al., 2018).

There are several other key details to consider when splinting including the fact that manufactured splints should be cared for as if they were custom-made for every client. Neoprene splints should be made specifically to fit each client. Other materials may require sewing or additional care. Circumferential splint designs are precise because they cover the entire body part. Single surface splints only cover one surface of the body part being positioned.

Arm Support Devices

Arm support devices are usually positioned overhead and are connected above the head via a line and attached to the wheelchair. People use suspension arm devices for many different reasons:

- Position the shoulder girdle
- Assists with gravity eliminated exercise
- Suggests exercise activity to improve ROM with repetition
- Platform for painful shoulders
- Provides a base for edema filled hands, above the heart
- Prohibits decrease of shoulder ROM

Mobile arm supports are specialized devices that balance the weight of the upper extremity and assist with shoulder and elbow motions via a ball-bearing joint (15). Other names for mobile arm support include the following:

- Ball-bearing feeder
- Ball-bearing arm support
- Balanced forearm orthosis
- Arm positioner

Mobile arm supports are used to decrease pain in upper limbs and used to improve upper limb function for people who present with serious arm paralysis:

- Spinal cord injury
- Muscular dystrophy
- Guillain-Barre syndrome
- Amyotrophic lateral sclerosis
- Poliomyelitis
- Polymyositis

Mobile arm supports assist arm motion facilitating active ROM in the shoulder and elbows. MAS also assist weak muscles that are unable to complete movement to participate in occupational performance. MAS allow for hand placement in multiple positions for occupational performance. MAS use the technical principles of gravity to assist limp muscles, provide balance to decrease the workload on limp muscles, and decrease shearing forces via ball-bearing joints.

References

American Occupational Therapy Association. (2014). Occupational therapy practice framework: Domain and process (3rd ed.). *American Journal of Occupational Therapy, 68*(Suppl. 1), S1–S51.

Anderson, K. N., Anderson, L. E., & Glanze, W. D. (1994). *Mosby's medical, nursing, and allied health dictionary* (4th ed.). Mosby.

Hollister, A., & Giurintano, D. (1999). How joints move. In P. W. Brand & A. Hollister (Eds.). *Clinical mechanics of the hand* (3rd ed.). Mosby.

Pedretti, L. W., Pendleton, H. M. H., & Schultz-Krohn, W. (2018). *Pedretti's occupational therapy: Practice skills for physical dysfunction* (8th ed.). Elsevier.

van der Heide, L. A., Gelderblom, G. J., & de Witte, L. P. (2014). Dynamic arm supports: Overview and categorization of dynamic arm supports for people with decreased arm function. *Prosthetics and Orthotics International, 38*, 287–302.

SECTION VI
Neurological Conditions

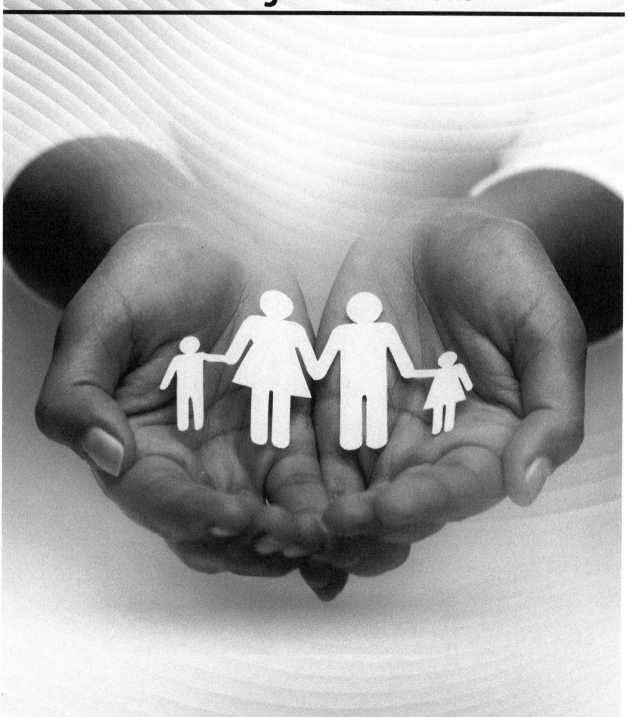

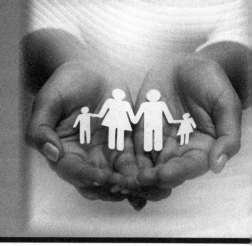

CHAPTER 12
Stroke and Occupational Therapy

Thousands of people are hospitalized each year, many of which secondary to cardiovascular issues. Stroke has been noted as the third leadin g cause of death secondary to heart disease and cancer (American Heart Association, 2015). Strokes are also called cerebrovascular accidents (CVA) and are an effect of lesions on the brain. Stroke is described as an early onset neurological abnormality of the vascular system that presents characteristics which correlate with involvement of the focal areas of the brain (World Health Organization, 2007). Strokes affect produce impairments on the opposite side of the brain of which the lesion appears. For example, if you have a stroke on the right side of your brain, you will see deficits on the left side of the body (Pedretti et al., 2018).

Types of Stroke

Strokes present in two ways: ischemic and hemorrhagic. Ischemic strokes are the result of poor blood flow to the brain due to a blockage or vessel constriction (American Heart Association, 2015; Bartels, 2016). Ischemic strokes are the most common. Embolisms are blood clots that travel from one body part to the brain or artery interrupting the perfusion of the brain. Hemorrhagic strokes are caused by bleeds via blood vessels within the subarachnoid and intracerebral layers of the brain. The most common causes for hemorrhagic strokes include the following:

- spontaneous lobar hemorrhage,
- arteriovenous malformation bleeding,
- ruptured saccular aneurysms, and
- deep hypertensive intracerebral hemorrhage (Kistler et al., 1994).

According to Pedretti, upper motor neuron damage produces hemiplegia, paralysis, sensory and visual disturbance, personality and cognitive changes. UMN dysfunction also produces speech and language disorders. In addition to UMN damage, other related syndromes present as a result of CVA. Cerebral anoxia and aneurysm can produce unilateral weakness. Transient ischemic attack (TIA) is a result of vascular disease of the brain secondary to a completed CVA. TIAs are identified by the mild, quiet, and continuous neurologic signs or symptoms which present abruptly, last for at least 24 hours, and fully resolve. TIAs have shown to be indicators for strokes and usually occur in people who have been diagnosed with atherosclerotic disease (American Heart Association, 2015). According to Pedretti, if a TIA develops secondary to extracranial vascular disease, surgery is necessary to renew vascularity. Carotid endarterectomy is the most surgical procedure used to restore blood flow following a CVA or a TIA and is effective in precluding resulting disability (Pedretti et al., 2018).

Strokes present as a result of cardiac sources like atrial-fibrillation (A-Fib), sinoatrial (SA) disorders, acute myocardial infarction (MI), endocarditis, cardiac tumors, and valve disorders. There are client factors for stroke that can be managed such as hypertension (HTN), cardiac disease, diabetes, smoking, alcohol abuse, drug abuse, and lifestyle traits (American Heart Association, 2015; Helgason & Wolf, 1997). Lifestyle traits can include weight, diet, exercise, and stress. Client factors that can lead to stroke and cannot be changed include age, race, gender, ethnicity, and heredity.

ISCHEMIC AND HEMORRHAGIC STROKE

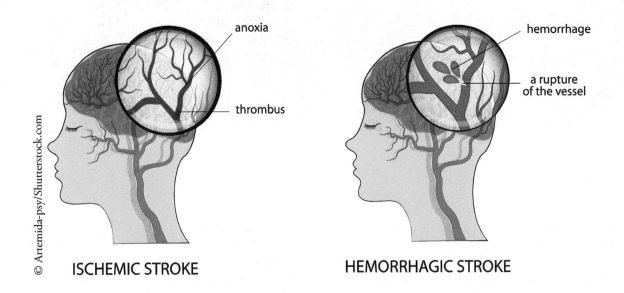

ISCHEMIC STROKE   HEMORRHAGIC STROKE

© Artemida-psy/Shutterstock.com

Stroke Effects

Stroke effects depend on which area of the brain is supplied by the damaged artery. Healthcare professionals use several types of equipment to diagnose strokes. Examples include computed tomography (CT), magnetic resonance imaging (MRI), positron emission tomography (PET), and single-photon emission computed tomography (SPECT; Bartels, 2016). Data gathered using any of these types of equipment assist in identifying the location, size, and severity of lesions. When a stroke occurs and affects the middle cerebral artery it produces hemiplegia, hemianesthesia, and homonymous hemianopia. Dominant hemisphere strokes cause speech and language deficits like Broca's or Wernicke's aphasia. Broca's aphasia is a deficit in word-finding or expression, where Wernicke's aphasia is a cognitive processing deficit. The nondominant hemisphere of the brain would include frontal lobe deficits and cause euphoria. Other effects of right hemisphere involvement include visual perceptual dysfunction, unilateral neglect, dressing apraxia, and loss of topographic memory. When the internal carotid artery has been affected it is due to poor perfusion of collateral circulation, producing contralateral hemiplegia, homonymous hemianopia, and hemianesthesia.

Middle cerebral artery strokes are the most prominent type of strokes (Árnadóttir, 1990; Bartels, 2016; Bourbonnais & Vanden Noven, 1989). They result in contralateral hemiplegia with bigger vessel inclusion of the face, arms, and tongue. The neck and head turn toward the side where the lesion is located (Branch, 1987; Chusid, 1985). Anterior cerebral artery strokes result from complete occlusion of the ACA and result in more pronounced contralateral lower limb weakness as compared to the upper limbs. ACA strokes produce apraxia, cognitive changes (Árnadóttir, 2016; Bartels, 2016), primitive reflexes, and bowel/bladder incontinence. Posterior cerebral artery (PCA) strokes produce larger affected areas because it supplies the brainstem, occipital, and temporal lobes. This development in the PCA causes sensory deficits, motor loss, involuntary movements, visual deficits, and memory loss (Árnadóttir, 2016; Bartels, 2016; Chusid, 1985). According to Pedretti, the cerebellar artery system blockage results in ipsilateral ataxia, dysphagia, dysarthria, and contralateral hemiparesis (Árnadóttir, 2016; Bartels, 2016; Branch, 1987; Chusid, 1985). Other common deficits that present as a result of occlusion of the PCA include contralateral loss of pain, temperature sensitivity, and ipsilateral facial analgesia. Vertebrobasilar artery occlusion causes deficits in brainstem function which also results in sensory and motor dysfunction. Cerebellar dysfunction creates a loss of proprioception, hemiplegia, sensory interruption, and unilateral participation from cranial nerves III and XII.

Assessment

In occupational therapy practice, the assessment phase of the OT process includes identifying client-specific deficits and interventions to address those deficits. The top-down approach to occupational therapy intervention begins with identifying client roles and their meanings (Trombly, 1993). Have the client explain what their life was like before the stroke (Trombly, 1993). It is the responsibility of the OT to connect the client's occupational performance, physical, and occupational parts of the intervention plan (Trombly, 1993).

Evaluation

The initial step in the evaluation process is completing a chart review. Next, explain occupational therapy's role in the rehabilitation process, ensure that the client understands their diagnosis and how you will assist them. Then, you select a client-centered assessment that identifies the specific deficits in occupational function (Law et al., 1995; Pollock, 1993). Give the client an opportunity to participate in the decision-making process (Law et al., 1995; Pollock, 1993). Be sure to use appropriate tools during the evaluation. Provide the client with a chance to reflect on their own performance and discuss individual goals (Law et al., 1995; Pollock, 1993). As occupational therapists we use activity analysis to select client factors and affected performance skills.

Functional Performance Limitations

Following a stroke, a person may present with several physical performance deficits that will affect their ability to live independently. Research has shown that core strength and control are precursors to ambulation, sitting balance, and ADL performance (Bohannon, 1995) (Franchignoni et al., 1997; Sandin & Smith, 1990). For example, poor safety awareness and a higher incidence of falls limit a person's ability to live independently (Gillen, 1998). Uncoordinated movement of the extremities also impairs a person's ability to interact with their environment safely (Gillen, 2016). Head and shoulder dysfunction can impair visual function and inhibit a person's ability to live alone. Other problems include decreased ADL and IADL performance (Gillen, 2016). Stroke effects on the torso or trunk present clinically as difficulty with lateral leaning and assuming static sitting postures that are not beneficial during the occupational performance. Torso and trunk effects following stroke also include spinal contractures, difficulty shifting weight through the pelvis, and trunk instability (Bohannon, 1995).

Interventions

Occupational therapy interventions for stroke rehabilitation include positioning the client in a neutral but active alignment during sitting. OTs use verbal cues, tactile cues, and visual cues as needed to guide the client through task performance. Other interventions for stroke can include dynamic sitting balance tasks, core strengthening, compensatory strategies, and home or environmental modifications.

Interventions for stroke ensuring that the client has a symmetrical base of support and midline position has been engaged. Allow the client to participate in weight-bearing activities to engage the upper and lower limbs. Occupational therapists can also modify or grade activities to encourage participation in daily living tasks. Optimal client position for seated tasks can be established as follows:

- Feet flat on the floor
- Bear weight equally through ischial tuberosities
- Pelvis in neutral
- Spine upright and midline
- Head and shoulders midline (Gillen, 2016)

Complications Following Stroke

Following a stroke, many complications can present and possibly inhibit the rehabilitation process, like subluxation. Subluxation is a partial dislocation of the shoulder joint. Skeletal muscle dysfunction, edema, muscle contractures, and overstretching the joint capsule are also possible complications following CVA (Bourbonnais & Vanden Noven, 1989; Gillen, 2016). Preventative measures for pain and contractures of unstable joints are important during the rehabilitation process. Soft tissue integrity, elongation, and length can lead to pain and discomfort

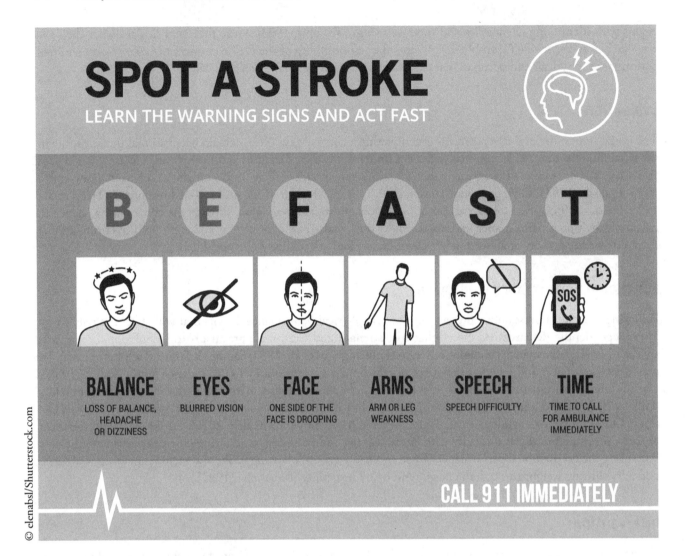

in the upper extremity. Positioning and stabilization of joints through splinting can also minimize damage to the surrounding tissue and protect the joint.

References

American Heart Association. (2015). Heart disease and stroke statistics: 2015 update. *Circulation, 131,* e29–e32.

Árnadóttir, G. (1990). *The brain and behavior: Assessing cortical dysfunction through activities of daily living.* Mosby.

Árnadóttir, G. (2016). Impact of neurobehavioral deficits of activities of daily living. In G. Gillen (Ed.), *Stroke rehabilitation: A function-based approach* (4th ed., pp. 376–426). Mosby.

Bartels, M. N. (2016). Pathophysiology, medical management and acute rehabilitation of stroke survivors. In G. Gillen (Ed.), *Stroke rehabilitation: A function-based approach* (4th ed., pp. 2–45). Mosby.

Bohannon, R. W. (1995). Recovery and correlates of trunk muscle strength after stroke. *International Journal of Rehabilitation Research, 18,* 162.

Bourbonnais, D., & Vanden Noven, S. (1989). Weakness in patients with hemiparesis. *American Journal of Occupational Therapy, 43,* 313.

Branch, E. F. (1987). The neuropathology of stroke. In P. W. Duncan & M. B. Badke (Eds.), *Stroke rehabilitation: The recovery of motor control.* Year Book.

Chusid, J. (1985). *Correlative neuroanatomy and functional neurology* (19th ed.). Lange.

Franchignoni, F. P., Tesio, L., Ricupero, C., & Martino, M. T. (1997). Trunk control test as an early predictor of stroke rehabilitation outcome. *Stroke, 28,* 1382–1385.

Gillen, G. (1998). Trunk control: A prerequisite to functional independence. In G. Gillen & A. Burkhardt (Eds.), *Stroke rehabilitation: A function-based approach* (pp. 69–89). Mosby.

Gillen, G. (2016). Trunk control: Supporting functional independence. In G. Gillen (Ed.), *Stroke rehabilitation: A function-based approach* (4th ed., pp. 360–393). Mosby.

Helgason, C. M., & Wolf, P. A. (1997). *American Heart Association Prevention Conference IV: Prevention and rehabilitation of stroke*. American Heart Association.

Kistler, J. P., Ropper, A. H., & Martin, J. B. (1994). Cerebrovascular disease. In K. J. Isselbacher et al. (Eds.), *Harrison's principles of internal medicine* (p. 29). McGraw-Hill.

Law, M., Baptiste, S., & Mills, J. (1995). Client-centered practice: What does it mean and does it make a difference? *Canadian Journal of Occupational Therapy, 62*, 250.

Pollock, N. (1993). Client-centered assessment. *American Journal of Occupational Therapy, 47*, 298.

Pedretti, L. W., Pendleton, H. M. H., & Schultz-Krohn, W. (2018). *Pedretti's occupational therapy: Practice skills for physical dysfunction* (8th ed.). Elsevier.

Sandin, K. J., & Smith, B. S. (1990). The measure of balance in sitting in stroke rehabilitation prognosis. *Stroke, 21*, 82.

Trombly, C. A. (1993). Anticipating the future: Assessment of occupational function. *American Journal of Occupational Therapy, 47*, 253.

World Health Organization. (2007). *International classification of diseases* (ICD-10). Author.

CHAPTER 13

Traumatic Brain Injury

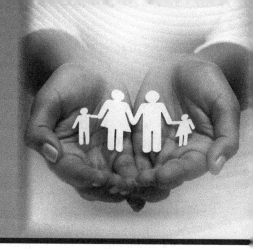

According to Pedretti, traumatic brain injury (TBI) is defined as damage to brain tissue due to external forces, usually mechanical, which lead to decreased levels of consciousness, post-traumatic amnesia, skull fractures, and other neurological developments related the trauma based on the findings, mental or physical evaluations (Ghajar, 2000; Sosin et al., 1996; Thurman, 1995). The Centers for Disease Control and Prevention reports that 5.3 million Americans currently have a chronic need for assistance when completing ADLs secondary to TBI (Brain Injury Association, 2006). The etiology of TBI corresponds with age. Children who are younger than 5 suffer injuries related to falls, car accidents, and physical abuse. Children of ages 5 to 15 suffer injuries secondary to bicycle accidents, skateboards, and horseback riding. Americans aged 15 to 40 suffer injury due to high-speed car accidents or motorcycle accidents. Young men aged 40 to 60 are 1.5 times more likely to develop a TBI than women. The age groups with the highest risk for TBI are 0 to 4-year olds and 15 to 19-year olds (Brain Injury Association, 2006). The geriatric population are injured secondary to falls or car accident involving a pedestrian (Englander & Cifu, 2003; Langlois et al., 2003). Among military personnel blasts are the leading cause of TBI on active duty (Brain Injury Association, 2006).

Concussion

Concussions are injuries to the brain caused by direct blows to the head, falls, or any act that produces a quick forward and backward motion of the head. Symptoms of concussions include headaches, lightheaded feeling, blurred vision, decreased memory, poor safety awareness and problem-solving, and alterations in coordination. Symptoms of concussion last for multiple days or months following the injury. Long-term effects of concussions present as poor attention or nerve and brain damage. Some people who have suffered multiple concussions can display very aggressive behavior and become violent. Cognitive-behavioral therapy can be of use for these clients. Chronic traumatic encephalopathy is progressive in nature and often occurs in people with a history of multiple brain injuries including concussions and sub-concussions (Mayo Clinic, n.d.). People who suffer from concussions display symptoms like decreased memory, confusion, depression, and aggression. TBI has been linked to substance abuse and there is a very high correlation between the two (Kraus et al., 1989).

Types of TBI

Non-TBI can be caused by drug toxicity or overdose, long-term substance abuse, carbon monoxide poisoning, or exposure to harmful chemicals. Other causes for non-TBI include

- Anoxia due to near-drowning or cardiopulmonary arrest
- Brain abscess
- Meningitis
- Encephalitis due to bacteria
- AIDS

- HIV
- Genetic or congenital disorders
- Chronic epilepsy
- Degenerative changes like dementia

The pathophysiology for primary and secondary prevention of TBI is categorically different. Primary prevention includes individual methods such as wearing a seatbelt, helmet, airbags, and roadside barrier use. Secondary prevention starts at the first responder contact with those who arrive on the accident scene first. TBI injuries normally develop as a result of primary focal and diffuse brain injuries (Pedretti et al., 2018). The causes of TBI are varied. A focal brain injury is the result of a direct impact with the head and an outside force or object, piercing injury due to a weapon, and impact of the brain with inner layers of the skull. Multifocal and diffuse brain injuries occur as a result of abrupt deceleration of the body and head with multiple forces supplied via the surface and subsequent areas of the brain. Intracerebral hemorrhage (ICH) occurs as a result of penetrating wounds and is common after falls or attacks. Subarachnoid hemorrhage (SAH) also referred to as intraventricular hemorrhage occurs when the arachnoid or pia mater layers of the brain are torn. Diffuse axonal injuries are defined as prototypic lesions on the brain due to abrupt deceleration. The extent of the injuries is determined by the duration and length of time the coma persists (Langlois et al., 2003). Secondary injuries occur as the result of swelling of the brain in a confined area such as the skull, poor blood flow, poor oxygen delivery to healthy and injured tissue.

TBI can also cause post-traumatic seizures and they are classified as "immediate" when they occur within the first 24 hours following an injury. Seizures are classified as "early" when they occur during the first 7 days following the injury. The seizures are classified as "late" after the first 7 days.

OT Intervention

OT intervention after a TBI should be directed on cognitive, behavioral, and occupational performance factors. Because TBI alters levels of consciousness OT intervention varies based on the severity of the coma. Coma scales measure how alert or aware a person is following a TBI. Many factors influence how a person will progress following a TBI. These factors include age, extent of the injury, medical, therapeutic, and environmental regulation. Pedretti describes consciousness as a state of environmental and self-awareness. Comas are defined as the loss of self-awareness and environmental awareness despite the outside influences.

The Glasgow Coma Scale (GCS) is the most common scale of measurement of comas used by healthcare professionals (Rosenthal, 1984). The GCS is scored in three categories:

- Eye-opening: 1 to 4 (Rosenthal, 1984)
- Best motor: 1 to 6 (most reliable; Rosenthal, 1984)
- Verbal response: 1 to 5 (speaking; Rosenthal, 1984)

Ranchos Los Amigos Scale of Cognitive Function is a measurement tool that describes levels of awareness and cognitive function. This scale is useful when training family and staff on behavioral interventions for clients.

Clinical Presentation for TBI

Many people suffer with altered patterns of function and mental changes as a result of TBI. Motor deficits are common with TBI and present themselves as follows:

- Decerebrate rigidity-extensor tone
- Decorticate rigidity-flexion tone
- Bruxism—teeth grinding
- Spasticity—velocity-dependent resistance
- Parkinsonism—velocity-independent resistance
- Torticollis—abnormal tone in the neck
- Myoclonus—involuntary jerky movements

- Tremor—involuntary rhythmic spasms
- Dystonia—slow writing, distal limb movements
- Athetosis—slow movements of the face and tongue
- Chorea—involuntary jerky movements without rhythm
- Hemiballismus—sudden irregular movements of flinging nature
- Tics—automated movements or vocalizations
- Pseudobulbar athetoid syndrome—abnormal postural tone

Post stroke spasticity of left lower extremity

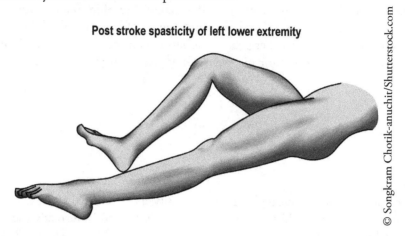

© Songkram Chotik-anuchit/Shutterstock.com

The cognitive status of those people who suffer from TBI varies depending on the type and location of the injury. Some common cognitive injuries include attention and concentration deficits, poor memory, poor task initiation, and termination. Clients also present with poor safety awareness and poor judgment, impulsive behavior, and poor executive function.

Perception is a deficit in which an inability to gauge or interpret environmental influences exists. Perceptual deficits are frequently the result of right hemisphere injury but can also occur in the left hemisphere. Perception is also categorized into the following groups:

- Visual perception
- Body schema perception
- Motor perception
- Speech and language perception

Other visual perceptual deficits may appear like:

- Figure-ground—ability to distinguish same-colored items from the same-colored backgrounds
- right/left discrimination—distinguish the right side from the left side
- form constancy—steady visualization of objects
- position in space—proprioception
- topographic orientation—location of objects or people

Other perceptual deficits present clinically as aphasia either Broca's or Wernicke's which are speech and language deficits. Dyslexia is a reading disturbance and agraphia is a writing disorder. Some clients suffer from dyscalculia which is a calculation disorder. Dysprosody is an impairment in the word-formation or understanding of the tonal inflections in speech. Occupational therapists should identify alternative means of communication for clients with perceptual disorders such as communication boards, notes, and hand gestures or sign language. Motor deficits are also common such as motor planning and apraxia. Ideational apraxia presents as the incapacity to understand the demands of a task or use the incorrect motor plan for a specific task. Ideomotor apraxia is the loss of kinetic memory for a unique task. Constructional apraxia presents clinically as the incapacity to correctly organize pieces to build a three-dimensional whole object.

Cognitive Deficits and TBI

According to Pedretti, psychosocial factors affect client's overall quality of life. Depression and withdrawal are common and often present together. Clients who are non-verbal can express themselves through body language to allow OTs to assess their moods. A client's self-concept is best described as a person's ability to identify humans by sex and gender, body image, strengths and limitations, and familial hierarchy, peer groups, and community engagement.

Social roles were developed through self-concept and are composed of intimate relationships with other people, feeling secluded or abandoned. Independent living situations are frequently sacrificed as a result of TBI, forcing the client to feel more dependent on other people and less in control of themselves. Many people suffer TBI and often lose loved ones as a result of a traumatic event. Grief presents itself in five stages:

- Denial
- Anger
- Bargaining
- Depression
- Acceptance

Affective changes include depression, increased emotional lability, and decreased effect due to neurological injury. Behavioral status refers to the Ranchos Los Amigos cognitive level IV and is normally the "frustrated" and "perplexed" levels. Clients who suffer from these symptoms are normally impulsive and agitated. They often yell, curse, snatch, or bite at other people secondary to their injury. Goals to address these behaviors should include providing a safe environment for all parties involved. Make sure that everyone is consistent with behavior techniques, decrease the use of restrictive modalities, and create an environment conducive to occupational participation. Other interventions for behaviors can include one on one coaching, psychotropic medications, and individualized behavior management plans. Environmental changes may be necessary including cubicle or net bed, alarms, helmets, and communication devices.

Post stroke spasticity of right upper extremity

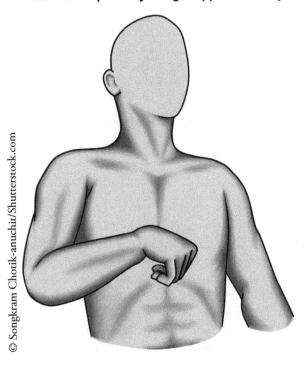

© Songkram Chotik-anuchit/Shutterstock.com

Evaluation

Evaluation of lower level TBI begins with short sessions at different times during the day. The environment should be quiet and allow for minimal distractions; this will improve the client's ability to hear and complete instructions. The first step in the evaluation process is to assess the level of alertness, sequencing, verbal participation, meaningful movement. Assess the level of arousal and vision. Sensation should be assessed next to identify responses to outside influences like pain, temperature, and joint movement. Joint range of motion is assessed to identify decorticate or decerebrate rigidity, spasticity, contractures, or heterotrophic ossification. Dysphagia is a condition in which a client cannot swallow or has difficulty with the swallow. Occupational therapists can assist with the hand-to-mouth portion of feeding and functional grasp. Lower level TBI evaluation should also include wheelchair positioning, bed positioning, sensory stimulation, and splinting. Evaluation of higher level TBI starts with the level of arousal and verbal responses. Cognition assessment includes sequencing, attention without distraction, and safety awareness. Perception is the next to be assessed and then ADL performance.

References

Brain Injury Association. (2006). *Fact sheets*. Author.

Englander, J., & Cifu, D. X. (1999). The older adult with traumatic brain injury. In M. Rosenthal, E. R. Griffith, J. S. Kreutzer, & B. Pentland (Eds.), *Rehabilitation of the adult and child with traumatic brain injury*. F. A. Davis.

Ghajar, J. (2000). Traumatic brain injury. *Lancet, 356*, 923.

Mayo Clinic. (n.d.). http://www.mayoclinic.org/diseases-conditions/chronic-traumatic-encephalopathy/basics/definition/con-20113581

Kraus, J. F., Morgenstern, H., Fife, D., Conroy, C., & Nourjah, P. (1989). Blood alcohol tests, prevalence of involvement, and outcomes following brain injury. *American Journal of Public Health, 79*, 294.

Langlois, J. A., Kegler, S. R., Butler, J. A., Gotsch, K. E., Johnson, R. L., Reichard, A. A., Webb, K. W., Coronado, V. G., Selassie, A. W., & Thurman, D. J. (2003). Traumatic brain injury–related hospital discharges: Results from a 14-state surveillance system, 1997. *MMWR Surveillance Summaries, 52* (4), 1–20.

Pedretti, L. W., Pendleton, H. M. H., & Schultz-Krohn, W. (2018). *Pedretti's occupational therapy: Practice skills for physical dysfunction* (8th ed.). Elsevier.

Rosenthal, M. (1984). Strategies for intervention with families of brain-injured patients. In B. A. Edelstein & E. T. Couture (Eds.), *Behavioral assessment and rehabilitation of the traumatically brain-damaged. Applied clinical psychology*. Springer. https://doi.org/10.1007/978-1-4757-9392-5_7

Sosin, D. M., Sniezek, J. E., & Thurman, D. J. (1996). Incidence of mild and moderate brain injury in the United States, 1991. *Brain Injury, 10*, 47.

Thurman, D. J. (1995). *Guidelines for surveillance of central nervous system injury*. Centers for Disease Control and Prevention.

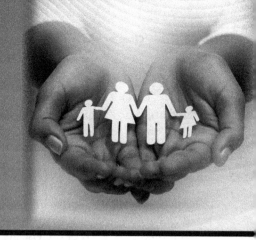

CHAPTER 14
Neurodegenerative Diseases of the Central Nervous System

Occupational therapists observe many diseases that affect the central nervous system many of which are degenerative and have lifelong effects (Gelb, 2005). Neurodegenerative disorders are described as disease processes that originate from defects in the body's neurological function and result in a constant decline in physical and/or cognitive changes that last for a lifetime. When a client's self-reliance becomes vulnerable, they decline in other areas of self-care (Schwartz et al., 1996). In this chapter we will discuss several neurodegenerative disorders including amyotrophic lateral sclerosis (ALS), Alzheimer's disease, Huntington's disease (HD), and multiple sclerosis (MS). Amyotrophic lateral sclerosis (ALS) or Lou Gehrig's disease (Belsh & Schiffman, 1996) is a set of neurologically progressive diseases that were on the body's motor neurons located inside the spinal column, brainstem, and primary motor cortex (ALS Continuing Education Module; Sorenson & Thurman, 2018). Several propositions for the development of ALS have been presented including motor neuron damage, genetic changes, metabolic disorders, metal toxicity, and viral infections (ALS Continuing Education Module; Sorenson & Thurman, 2018). ALS primarily causes deficits to the upper motor neurons which produce weakness, spasticity, and increased reflex response. Damage to lower motor neurons produces weakness and muscle wasting in the limbs. ALS starts as focal weakness in the upper extremities, lower extremities, or bulbar muscles and progresses quickly. The pathophysiology of ALS is undetermined. Many people who present with ALS die within 3–5 years secondary to respiratory problems. ALS occurs more frequently in men than women. Lou Gehrig's disease has no effect on eye function, bowel or bladder function, or sensory function (ALS Continuing Education Module; Sorenson & Thurman, 2018). According to Pedretti, there are currently three forms of ALS:

- **Sporadic—most common and affects 90% to 95% of people**
- **Familial—occurs more than once in a family lineage**
- **Guamanian—very high occurrence in Guam and the Trust Territories of the Pacific in the 1950s**

ALS can also produce effects that present clinically as progressive bulbar palsy, which damages the corticobulbar tracts and brainstem motor nuclei. Symptoms appear as dysarthria, dysphagia, facial and tongue weakness, and muscle wasting (Kim et al., 2009; National Institute of Neurological Disorders and Stroke). Another disease process that is closely related to ALS is progressive spinal muscular atrophy which is the result of lower motor neuron damage in the brain and spinal cord (Kim et al., 2009; National Institute of Neurological Disorders and Stroke). Progressive spinal muscular atrophy produces symptoms such as muscle

Amyotrophic Lateral Sclerosis (ALS)

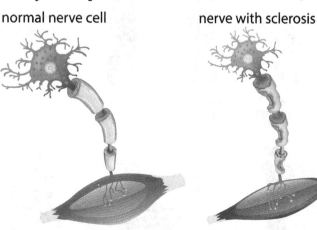

normal nerve cell

nerve with sclerosis

muscle contracts

muscle unable to contract

© BlueRingMedia/Shutterstock.com

atrophy of the extremities, trunk, and occasionally bulbar muscles (Kim et al., 2009; National Institute of Neurological Disorders and Stroke). The last associated disease process is primary lateral sclerosis which is the result of upper motor neuron damage and corticospinal and corticobulbar regions. Symptoms include progressive spastic paraparesis (Kim, et al., 2009; National Institute of Neurological Disorders and Stroke).

ALS stages and Intervention Strategies

There are six clinical presentation stages for ALS (Yase, 1972). In the first stage the client can walk and has no deficits with ADL performance with mild muscle weakness. During the initial stage activity levels are normal and moderate levels of exercise are appropriate. In the second stage the client remains ambulatory with moderate muscle weakness and more fatigue. Activity levels at stage II moderate exercise minimal lifestyle changes, and some active assistive activities. Clients' equipment needs at this stage include hands-free devices, tablets, and assistive devices. In the third stage the client can still walk, has severe muscle weakness, difficulty with ADL performance, and increased fatigue. Activity levels include active assistive exercise, home modifications, and joint pain management. Equipment needs include the use of smart technology, adaptive devices, home and environmental modifications. Stage four of ALS presents as completely dependent in lower extremities with severe weakness in the lower extremity and dependent with most ADL tasks. Activities include a passive range of motion with moderate exercise levels. Equipment needs include smart technology and home modifications. Stages 5 and 6 clients are completely dependent with ADLs and mobility, passive range of motion, pain management, prevention of skin breakdown. Equipment needs for these stages include smart technology and environmental modifications.

ALS Evaluation

Occupational therapy evaluation begins with assessing the client's ADL and IADL performance. Evaluation of executive function and cognitive dysfunction should also be included (Raaphorst et al., 2010). Observe the client

Amyotrophic Lateral Sclerosis (ALS)

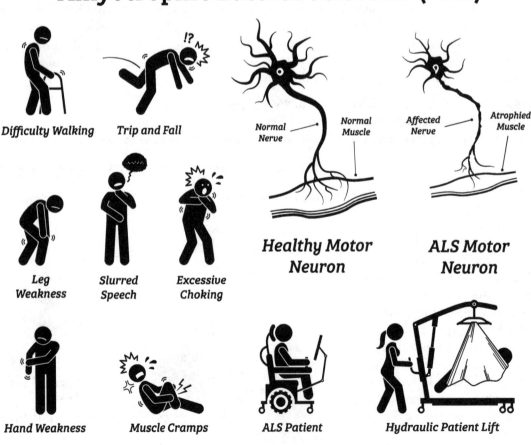

Difficulty Walking   Trip and Fall   Normal Nerve   Normal Muscle   Affected Nerve   Atrophied Muscle

Leg Weakness   Slurred Speech   Excessive Choking   **Healthy Motor Neuron**   **ALS Motor Neuron**

Hand Weakness   Muscle Cramps   ALS Patient   Hydraulic Patient Lift

© Leremy/Shutterstock.com

for behavioral dysfunction that can affect their ability to complete daily living tasks (Allen et al., 1992). Include the client's family or caregiver throughout the evaluation process and as the disease advances. Be sure to consider social, cultural, and religious beliefs when planning interventions and training for caregivers. Recommend any psychosocial resources that may be available to the client or caregivers in the local area. Support groups and caregiver burn out seminars are also available virtually and in the traditional setting.

Alzheimer's Disease

Alzheimer's disease is a progressive degenerative dysfunction of the brain. Alzheimer's disease is also known as dementia, which is the umbrella term for this type of disorder. The most common form of dementia is Alzheimer's disease and is diagnosed in people over the age of 65. The main symptom of Alzheimer's disease is decreased short-term memory that declines over time, minimum of one cognitive deficit such as apraxia, aphasia, agnosia, or poor executive function. There are three types of dementia:

- **Vascular dementia—the blood perfusion to the brain is poor causing poor reasoning, planning, and judgment** (Mayo Foundation for Medical Education and Research, 2020)
- **Lewy Body dementia—protein-specific deposits affecting thinking, memory, and movement** (Mayo Foundation for Medical Education and Research, 2020)
- **Frontotemporal dementia—deficits affect the frontal and temporal lobes of the brain** (Mayo Foundation for Medical Education and Research, 2020)

Alzheimer's disease is classified as a mental disorder and the cause is not known (American Psychological Association, 2013). The life expectancy is approximately 8–10 years that is dependent on the rate of progression. Healthcare professionals use the Global Deterioration Scale (GDS) to measure cognitive function for those people who suffer from degenerative dementia. The GDS is broken down into seven stages. Stages 1 to 3 are pre-dementia stages and stages 4 to 7 are dementia stages. Alzheimer's disease has several other clinical presentations such as altered behavior, mood disturbance, delirium deficits, poor attention span, poor alertness, and impaired perception.

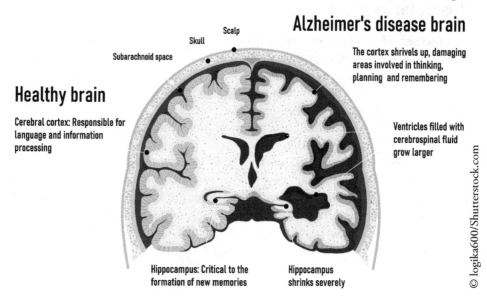

Alzheimer's Disease Evaluation

Occupational therapy evaluation begins with a functional assessment based on the client's cognitive function (Birnesser, 1997). OTs should include any issues and monitoring the caregiver is crucial; however, watching the caregiver complete the task is important (Birnesser, 1997). The assessment should examine the executive function of clients who present with symptoms of dementia (Birnesser, 1997). The Kitchen Task Assessment is used to measure the level of support a person who has senile dementia will need based on the completion of a cooking task

(Baum & Edwards, 1993a, 1993b). The Allen Cognitive Level determines how well a client solves problems while participating in a perceptual-motor task (Allen, 1991). The Assessment of Motor Process Skills measures motor and process skills using task performance in IADLs (Fisher, 1991).

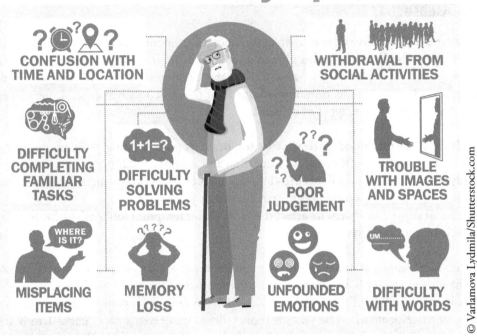

Alzheimer's Disease Intervention

Occupational therapists should aim interventions at maintaining the cognitive function that remains following a diagnosis of Alzheimer's disease (American Psychiatric Association, 1994; Atchison, 1994; Hasselkus, 1998; Joiner & Hansel, 1996). Develop an intervention plan that is structured and includes supervision as needed throughout the process. Dementia progresses differently for each person and allowing for modifications along the way will enhance the client's adjustment to a new role identity.

Occupational therapy intervention should be directed at improving the functional capacity of a client with Alzheimer's disease by constantly modifying ADL tasks and changing the physical and social surroundings during the diseases' progression (Baum, 1991). OT goals are focused on decreasing behavior dysfunction, improving function and independence. Another very important goal is to create a safe environment. The final overall goal of OT intervention for Alzheimer's disease is to supply services that improve strong qualities that are still intact. Other goals can include minimizing caregiver burnout and maintaining the client in the least restrictive environment (Li R, et al. 2014). Providing caregiver support during the intervention process is important to minimize stress and to assist caregivers with developing strategies to cope with being a caregiver (Baum, 1991).

Huntington's Disease

Huntington's disease is a neurological progressive disease that affects voluntary and involuntary movements. Huntington's disease has a 50% probability to be transmitted from parents to offspring. The corpus striatum and the breakdown of the caudate nucleus are associated with the development of Huntington's disease (Cicchetti & Parent, 1996; Parent & Cicchetti, 1998). The corpus striatum is essential to motor control and damage to this area of the brain accounts for the development of chorea-like movements (Cicchetti & Parent, 1996; Parent & Cicchetti, 1998). The caudate nucleus has been connected to cognitive and emotional functions along with the cerebral cortex (Cicchetti & Parent, 1996; Parent & Cicchetti, 1998).

HUNTINGTON'S DISEASE

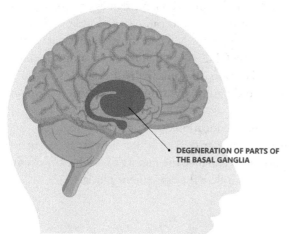

DEGENERATION OF PARTS OF THE BASAL GANGLIA

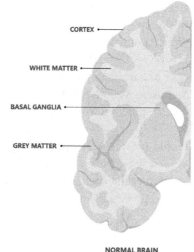

CORTEX

WHITE MATTER

BASAL GANGLIA

GREY MATTER

NORMAL BRAIN   HUNTINGTON'S DISEASE BRAIN

© rumruay/Shutterstock.com

Huntington's disease presents in three stages (Walker, 2007): (1) Early stage presents as chorea movements which are described as fast, involuntary, and uncoordinated movements (159). Chorea only presents in the hands and is absent during sleep (Walker, 2007; Wiederholt, 2000). (2) Middle stage presents as disturbances in memory and executive function. Other clinical symptoms include the poor transfer of learning, difficulty with ambulation, and dysphagia (Folstein et al., 1975). Bradykinesia and akinesia are also common symptoms of Huntington's disease. Clients also demonstrate difficulty with participating in purposeful activities, understanding oral instruction, and chorea worsens. Suicide is common among people diagnosed with Huntington's disease (Walker, 2007; Wiederholt, 2000). (3) Late stage presents with hypertonicity and rigidity instead of chorea (Walker, 2007; Wiederholt, 2000). There is a severe decline in voluntary movement and deficits with eye movement occur (Penney & Young, 1998). This stage will require long-term care assistance.

According to Pedretti, occupational therapy intervention is aimed at addressing cognitive deficits including memory and concentration. Develop a daily schedule and create lists to manage tasks efficiently. Other occupational therapy interventions include problem-solving (Cruickshank et al., 2015) and workplace accommodations. Using electronic planners or organizers can improve a client's function in the workplace. Providing a quiet work environment and decreasing the number of external stimuli can also enhance a client's ability to perform workplace tasks successfully. Psychological deficits that appear during the early stage include anxiety, depression, and irritability (Folstein, 1989; Hayden, 1996). Encourage the client to continue to participate in social engagements and purposeful activities are essential for the client with Huntington's disease (Phillips, 1982).

Multiple Sclerosis

Multiple sclerosis (MS) is a progressive and inflammatory neurological disease that is the result of damage to the myelin sheath in the CNS. Myelin is generally destroyed in uncommon regions of the white matter with the axon protected (Reidak et al., 2010). Interruption of the myelin sheath

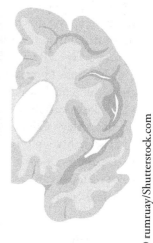

Normal   Multiple Sclerosis

Myelin sheath   Damaged myelin

© Alila Medical Media/Shutterstock.com

has altering effects on the axon length of the damaged portion of the nerve (Calabresi, 2004). Axons are the conduct impulse much slower due to inflammation of the myelin sheath. People who have damage to the myelin sheath demonstrate sensory deficits, uncoordinated movements, visual deficits, and muscle weakness. MS onset begins between 20 and 45 years of age (Reidak et al., 2010). There is no cure for MS and the disease is terminal.

The clinical presentation of MS is directly related to the part of the CNS affected. These symptoms include fatigue, unilateral weakness or numbness in the limbs, unilateral visual deficits, diplopia, pain or tingling sensation, shock-like sensations with cervical spine movement, tremors, poor coordination, dysarthria, and bowel or bladder function (Mayo Clinic, n.d.).

The evaluation process should include ADL and IADL performance, education, work, play, leisure, and social participation. Develop the occupational profile and establish performance criteria to assess functional independence with self-care tasks. Inclusion of the client caregiver is important to enhance the quality of life for the client. Evaluate sleep patterns, perceptual processing, and visual function to complete the assessment phase.

Parkinson's Disease

Parkinson's disease (PD) is one of the most common neurologically degenerative diseases in the United States (Shulman et al., 2010). There are three trademark symptoms associated with PD. They are tremor, rigidity, and bradykinesia. PD is more common in adults over age 55 but it can present in people who are younger than 55 (de Rijk et al., 1995; Shulman et al., 2010). There is a higher rate of PD that occurs in men than women aged 55–74, after age 74 women have a rate of development for PD. The pathophysiology of PD has not been identified and there is no cure for PD. Genetics has been linked to the underlying cause of PD; no other indicators have been noted. The etiology of PD is connected to the substantia nigra in the brain (Olanow et al., 1998). The substantia nigra in conjunction with the pars compacta reduce the overall activity inside the basal ganglia which decreases the production of dopamine and which directly affects movement. The clinical presentation of PD is primarily movement-based and is not a fatal disease (Phillips & Stelmach, 1996). People who have been diagnosed with PD are more likely to develop pneumonia. PD has traits that present like voluntary and involuntary movements (Phillips & Stelmach, 1996). Clients often have difficulty with task initiation and slow movement during task completion. These symptoms have an impact on the performance of ADL tasks and functional independence with self-care completion. Rigidity and muscle stiffness are also symptoms of PD. Other symptoms present as balance deficits and decrease fine motor control.

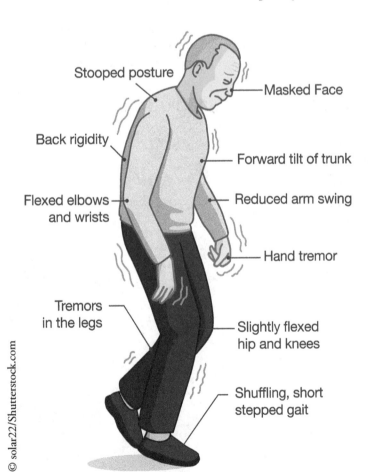

Parkinson's Disease Symptoms

- Stooped posture
- Masked Face
- Back rigidity
- Forward tilt of trunk
- Flexed elbows and wrists
- Reduced arm swing
- Hand tremor
- Tremors in the legs
- Slightly flexed hip and knees
- Shuffling, short stepped gait

© solar22/Shutterstock.com

PD Interventions

According to Pedretti, the level of OT services provided to clients will depend vastly on the severity of the PD diagnosis. Occupational therapists provide compensatory strategies, education, home modifications, and community-based resources. Always begin with the occupational profile and client-centered goals (Roger & Medved, 2010). Choose occupations that are of interest and important to the client. Identify any community-based resources for the client and their family. Home modifications are essential to improving safety and increasing a client's level of independent function, especially during feeding. In the middle stages of PD oral motor control becomes an issue. Dysphagia and excessive oral secretions can add to the social stigma associated with PD. OTs should incorporate oral motor exercises to improve self-feeding. The tremors can be addressed using built-up handles and medication. Other home modifications include removal of any fall hazards and the addition of adaptive equipment like grab bars. Alterations in clothing fasteners and slip-on shoes should be implemented early on during the disease course. Incorporate exercise into the client's daily routine to improve strength and posture. As PD progresses the client will require more assistance with self-care tasks. During the final stage of PD, the client will be overcome with the motor deficits associated with the progression of the disease like tremors and rigidity making it impossible to perform self-care tasks independently (Hoehn, 1967). Psychosocial issues become the more prevalent like depression can be addressed with community resources and coping strategies. The use of voice activated and smart technology should be used to allow the client control over their environment.

References

Allen C. (1991). *Allen Cognitive Level (ACL) test.* American Occupational Therapy Foundation.

Allen, C. K., Earhart, C. A., & Blue, T. (1992). *Occupational therapy treatment goals for the physically and cognitively disabled.* American Occupational Therapy Association.

Alzheimer's Association. (n.d.). *10 early signs and symptoms of Alzheimer's.* http://www.alz.org/10-signs-symptoms-alzheimers-dementia.asp

American Psychiatric Association. (1994). *Diagnostic and statistical manual of mental disorders* (4th ed.). Author.

American Psychological Association. (2013). *Diagnostic and statistical manual of mental disorders* (5th ed.). Author.

Atchison, P. (1994). Helping people with Alzheimer's and their families preserve independence. *OT Week, 8,* 16.

Baum, C. (1991). Addressing the needs of the cognitively impaired elderly from a family policy perspective. *American Journal of Occupational Therapy, 45,* 594.

Baum, C., & Edwards, D. (1993a). Identification and measurement of productive behaviors in senile dementia of the Alzheimer's type. *Gerontologist, 33,* 403.

Baum, C., & Edwards, D. (1993b). Cognitive performance in senile dementia of Alzheimer's type: The Kitchen Task Assessment. *American Journal of Occupational Therapy, 47,* 5.

Belsh, J. M., & Schiffman, P. L. (1996). The amyotrophic lateral sclerosis (ALS) patient perspective on misdiagnosis and its repercussions. *Journal of the Neurological Sciences, 139*(Suppl.), 110–116. https://doi.org/10.1016/0022-510x(96)00088-3

Birnesser, L. (1997). Treating dementia: Practical strategies for long-term care. *OT Practice, 2,* 16.

Calabresi, P. A. (2004). Diagnosis and management of multiple sclerosis. *American Family Physician, 70*(10), 1935–1944.

Cicchetti, F., & Parent, A. (1996). Striatal interneurons in Huntington's disease: Selective increase in the density of calretinin-immunoreactive medium-sized neurons. *Movement Disorders, 11,* 619.

Cruickshank, T. M., Thompson, J. A., Domínguez J. F., Reyes, A. P., Bynevelt, M., Georgiou-Karistianis, N., Barker, R. A., & Ziman, M. R. (2015). The effect of multidisciplinary rehabilitation on brain structure and cognition in Huntington's disease: An exploratory study. *Brain Behavior, 5,* e00312.

de Rijk, M. C., Breteler, M. M. B., Graveland, G. A., Ott, A., Grobbee, D. E., van der Meche, F. G. A., & Hofman, A. (1995). Prevalence of Parkinson's disease in the elderly: The Rotterdam Study. *Neurology, 45,* 2143. doi:https://doi.org/10.1212/WNL.45.12.2143

Fisher, A. (1991). *The assessment of motor and process skill (AMPS) in assessing adults: Functional measures and successful outcomes.* American Occupational Therapy Foundation.

Folstein, M. F., Folstein, S. E., & McHugh, P. R. (1975). "Mini Mental State": A practical method for grading the cognitive state of patients for the clinician. *Journal of Psychiatric Research, 12,* 189–198.

Folstein, S. E. (1989). *Huntington's disease: A disorder of families.* Johns Hopkins University Press.

Gelb, D. J. (2005). *Introduction to clinical neurology* (3rd ed.). Elsevier.

Hasselkus, B. (1998). Occupation and well-being in dementia: The experience of day-care staff. *American Journal of Occupational Therapy, 52,* 423.

Hayden, M. R. (1996). *Huntington's chorea.* Springer-Verlag.

Hoehn, M. M., & Yahr, M. D. (1967). Parkinsonism: Onset, progression and mortality. *Neurology, 17,* 427.

Joiner, C., & Hansel, M. (1996). Empowering the geriatric client. *OT Practice, 1,* 34–39.

Kim, W-K., Liu, X., Sandner, J., Pasmantier, M., Andrews, J., Rowland, L. P., & Mitsumoto, H. (2009). Study of 962 patients indicates progressive muscular atrophy is a form of ALS. *Neurology, 73,* 1686–1692.

Li, R., Cooper, C., Barber, J., Rapaport, P., Griffin, M., & Livingston, G. (2014). Coping strategies as mediators of the effect of the START (strategies for RelaTives) intervention on psychological morbidity for family carers of people with dementia in a randomised controlled trial. *Journal of Affective Disorders, 168,* 298–305.

Mayo Clinic. (n.d.). *Diseases and conditions multiple sclerosis.* http://www.mayoclinic.org/diseases-conditions/multiple-sclerosis/basics/symptoms/con-20026689

Mayo Foundation for Medical Education and Research. (2020). *Alzheimer's Disease.* National Institute of Neurological Disorders and Stroke. http://scdn.prod-carehubs.net/n7-mcnn/7bcc9724adf7b803/uploads/2012/07/Alzheimers-Study.pdf

Olanow, C. W., Olanow, C. W., Jenner, P., Tatton, N. A., & Tatton, W. G. (1998). Neurodegeneration and Parkinson's disease. In J. Jankovic & E. Tolosa (Eds.), *Parkinson's disease and movement disorders* (3rd ed.). Williams & Wilkins.

Parent, A., & Cicchetti, F. (1998). The current model of basal ganglia organization under scrutiny. *Movement Disorders, 13,* 199.

Penney, J. B., & Young, A. B. (1998). Huntington's disease. In J. Jankovic & E. Tolosa (Eds.), *Parkinson's disease and movement disorders* (3rd ed.). Williams & Wilkins.

Pedretti, L. W., Pendleton, H. M. H., & Schultz-Krohn, W. (2018). *Pedretti's occupational therapy: Practice skills for physical dysfunction* (8th ed.). Elsevier.

Phillips, D. H. (1982). *Living with Huntington's disease.* University of Wisconsin Press.

Phillips, J. G., & Stelmach, G. E. (1996). Parkinson's disease and other involuntary movement disorders of the basal ganglia. In C. M. Fredericks & L. K. Saladin (Eds.), *Pathophysiology of the motor systems (pp. 424–444).* F. A. Davis.

Raaphorst, J., de Visser, M., Linssen, W. H. J. P., & de Haan, R. (2010). The cognitive profile of amyotrophic lateral sclerosis: A meta-analysis. *Amyotrophic Lateral Sclerosis and Frontotemporal Degeneration, 11,* 27–37.

Reidak, K., Jackson, S., & Giovannoni, G. (2010). Multiple sclerosis: A practical overview for clinicians. *British Medical Bulletin, 95,* 79–104.

Roger, K. S., & Medved, M. I. (2010). Living with Parkinson's disease: Managing identity together. *International Journal of Qualitative Studies on Health and Well-being, 30,* 5.

Schwartz, C. E., Coulthard-Morris, L., Zeng, Q., & Retzlaff, P. (1996). Measuring self-efficacy in people with multiple sclerosis: A validation study. *Archives of Physical Medicine and Rehabilitation, 77,* 394–398.

Shulman, J. M., DeJager, P. L., & Feany, M. B. (2010). Parkinson's disease: Genetics and pathogenesis. *Annual Review of Pathology, 6,* 193–222.

Sorenson, E., & Thurman, D. J. (2018). *Amyotrophic Lateral Sclerosis (ALS) Continuing Education Module.* http://www.atsdr.cdc.gov/emes/ALS

Walker, F. O. (2007). Huntington's disease. *Lancet, 369,* 218–228.

Wiederholt, W. (2000). Parkinson's disease and other movement disorders. *Neurology for non-neurologists* (4th ed.). W. B. Saunders.

Yase, Y. (1972). The pathogenesis of amyotrophic lateral sclerosis. *The Lancet, 300*(7772), 292–296.

SECTION VII
Spinal Cord Injuries

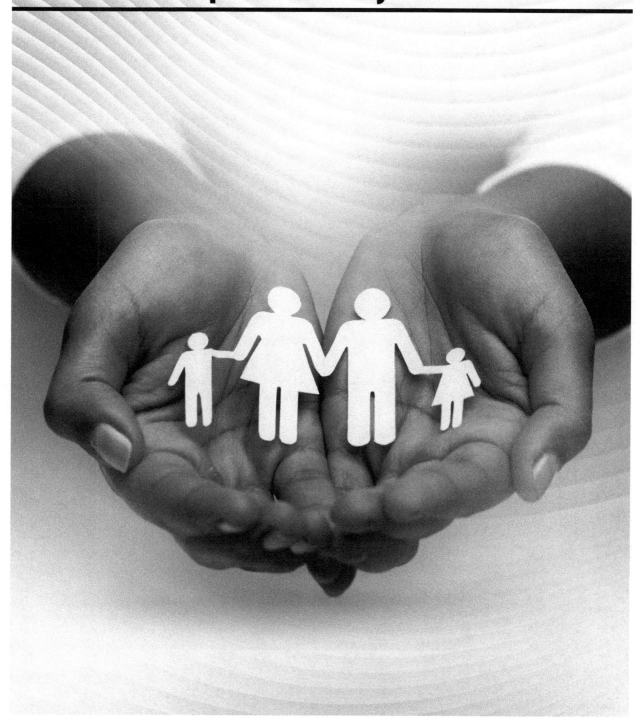

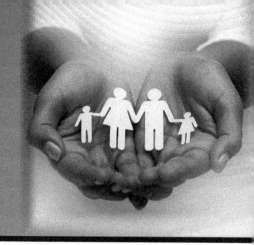

CHAPTER 15
Spinal Cord Injuries

Spinal cord injuries (SCI) vary according to the location and severity of the defect (Roberts et al., 2017). Spinal cord injuries are either labeled as complete or incomplete injuries. A complete injury is the total loss of movement and sensory function due to total blockage of the ascending and descending nerve tracts distal to the level of the injury. An incomplete injury is any degree of sensory or motor function that remains intact distal to the level of the injury. There are five classifications for spinal cord injuries and are labeled from A to E (Roberts et al., 2017). A being a complete injury and E being a normal functioning spinal cord (Roberts et al., 2017).

After an SCI people suffer from the spinal shock which can last up to 6 weeks. During spinal shock, reflexes are completely diminished and this is known as areflexia. During the period of areflexia, the bladder and bowel are flaccid. These dysfunctions are caused by a decline in the vasoconstriction of blood vessels, decreased blood pressure, bradycardia, and no sweating distal to the injury. Following an SCI, the cord itself is usually intact distal to the injury and the muscle innervation distal to the injury develops spasticity.

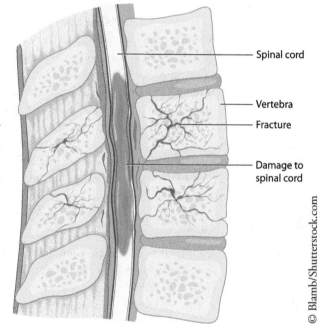

- Spinal cord
- Vertebra
- Fracture
- Damage to spinal cord

© Blamb/Shutterstock.com

Cord Syndromes

Central cord syndrome is the result of destroyed cells located in the center of the spinal cord and is the most common incomplete cord syndrome. Central cord syndrome causes increased sensory and motor deficits in the arms secondary to nerve tracts which are centrally located than the legs (McKinley et al., 2007; National Institute of Neurological Disorders and Stroke, 2014). *Brown-Sequard syndrome* occurs when only one side of the spinal cord is injured secondary to a penetrating injury or trauma. Distal to the level of the injury, there is a motor interruption, absence of proprioception on the injured side of the cord, and no pain response is present. *Anterior cord syndrome* occurs as a result of injury to the spinal artery or the front of the cord. Loss of motor function, pain, temperature, and sensation all affect proprioception. Proprioception is functional. *Cauda equina syndrome* occurs as the result of injury to peripheral nerves. Fractures are a common cause of Cauda equina syndrome distal to L2 level and produce hypotonic paralysis. People who suffer from Cauda equina syndrome receive a better outcome prognosis due to the ability of the peripheral to regenerate. *Conus Medullaris syndrome* results from damage to the sacral cord and lumbar nerve roots inside the neural canal. These injuries cause the loss of reflexes in the bladder, bowel, and legs.

The outcome prognosis for severe neuromuscular function and recovery is based on whether the injury is complete or incomplete (Grant et al., 2015; Kirshblum et al., 2007). If the motor function has not returned in 48 hours following the injury, then the likelihood that motor function would return is poor. Incomplete to complete function can be achieved and possibly happen during the initial 6 months following trauma. The motor function returns gradually to those people who suffer from incomplete injuries.

Spinal Stenosis

Spinal stenosis typically occurs due to arthritis that causes the spinal column to narrow and compresses the spinal cord. The spine is very delicate. It is made up of nerves that run through the vertebrae and conduct signals to the brain and the rest of the body. The process of spinal stenosis is steady and it can appear in the cervical, thoracic, lumbar, and sacrum part of the spine. If the narrowing is extensive, it can tamp the nerves and cause a vast volume of other symptoms which are sometimes misdiagnosed in a patient visit to the primary doctor. Lumbar spinal stenosis can cause bowel or bladder irregularities in the form of incontinence.

Lumbar spinal stenosis can be caused by aging and arthritis. Arthritis occurs when there is a breakdown of cartilage and the growth of bones. As the body ages, it goes through a degenerative process. Lumbar spinal stenosis will not cause any symptoms, but it will appear on an MRI or a CT scan. In order to diagnose this condition, a doctor will ask a few questions about your medical history and order an X-ray, MRI, or CT scan.

Ligamentum flavum gigantism can lead to constriction of the spinal canal. It is made of bands of elastic tissue that runs between the lamina from the axis to the sacrum, the ligamentum flavum connects the laminae and fuses with the facet joint capsules. These bands cover the spinal cord.

Occupational therapy is used to treat spinal stenosis. Patients complete functional tasks such as ADLs and IADL and participate in the therapeutic activity. Hot packs are used to help relax the muscles along the spine. Transcutaneous electrical nerve stimulation (TENS) unit along with medication such as Tylenol, Motrin, and Gabapentin are used to manage pain in lumbar spinal stenosis.

Medical Management

Immediately following an SCI, the cord should *not* be moved during the transfer from the accident site. First responders use a hard stretcher, with the client's head and shoulders strapped onto the board. Healthcare professionals prescribe anti-inflammatory agents after the injury. Surgery is completed to decompress the spinal cord, stabilize the cord, and achieve functional body position. SCI facilities are equipped with special equipment like special beds and other devices for those people who will be on bed rest for an extended time (Consortium for Spinal Cord Medicine, 2008). Clients are issued cervical collars or halo vests to help stabilize the spine during transfers (Ranchos Los Amigos National Rehabilitation Center). Evidence has shown that clients who attend rehabilitation programs experience greater functional improvements (Consortium for Spinal Cord Medicine, 2008; Juknis et al., 2012).

Complications

Clients who suffer a loss of sensation are at increased risk for developing skin breakdown. Increased pressure decreases the amount of blood in the area, resulting in necrosis. Necrosis is tissue death and requires sharp debridement or surgery to remedy. Heat modalities are contraindicated for people who have sensation impairment. Other complications for SCI include friction, which can damage tissue below the injury site. Clients with no sensation cannot feel the friction created during a transfer or change in position. Skin breakdown normally happens over bony prominences such as the ischium, sacrum, trochanters, elbows, and heels. Signs of skin compromise include redness in the area, skin blanches when pressed. These are indications of the initial stages of necrosis. Skin blisters develop in the area. Skin compromise can be prevented by alleviating pressure points and guarding susceptible areas against friction, moisture, and heat. Clients turn schedules, specialty mattresses, wheelchair seat cushions, stuffing or padding, and changes in position and minimize the potential for skin breakdown. Splints and orthosis can cause skin compromise, more frequently with decreased sensation.

Neurogenic bladder and bowel are caused by a disturbance in nerve function that controls the bowel and bladder. Clients cannot empty the bladder which results in urinary incontinence, urinary frequency, and bladder infections. Clients who suffer from a neurogenic bowel present with constipation, bowel incontinence, and fecal impaction. Clients with injuries at levels T12-L1 or higher will not control their bladder, which can also result in the spastic bladder.

Decreased vital capacity is a concern for people who have cervical or high thoracic injuries. These people have limited expansion in the chest and therefore the ability to cough is diminished due to paralysis or weakness in the diaphragm. Decreased vital capacity leads to respiratory infections and decreased activity tolerance. Training a client on how to perform energy conservation techniques via breathing.

Osteoporosis occurs as a result of extended nonuse of bones, specifically the legs. Pathological fractures often occur as secondary to osteoporosis. Areas that are most vulnerable to fractures are the supracondylar area of the femur, proximal tibia, and distal tibia, the intertrochanteric area of the femur, and the neck of the femur. Interventions for osteoporosis include standing tasks which can prolong the progression of the disease process.

Orthostatic hypotension occurs as a result of poor muscle tone in the abdomen which can cause blood to pool in the area, which results in poor blood flow. The condition is characterized by a decline of 10 mm Hg or higher in systolic blood pressure. Orthostatic hypotension develops when a client changes from supine to sit fast (Ditunno et al., 2012). The client appears dizzy, nauseous, and may faint. Intervention should begin with immediately returning the client to a reclined position and legs elevated. The secondary intervention begins with applying abdominal binders, compression garments, TED hose, and medications.

Autonomic Dysreflexia is a condition seen in people who suffer injury above T6 level. Autonomic dysreflexia develops because the autonomic nervous system is responding to influence such as bladder distension, fecal impaction, irritated bladder, rectal manipulation, thermal or painful stimulus, or visceral stimulus. Clinical signs and symptoms include severe headache, anxiety, sweating, chills, stuffy nose, hypertension, and slowed breathing (Consortium for Spinal Cord Injury, 1997; Kirshblum et al., 2011). This condition is life-threatening. The intervention begins with positioning the client upright and taking off any garments that limit movement or compression garments to decrease blood pressure. Assess if the client will need to have their bladder emptied or catheter examined for a blockage.

Spasticity happens in all people who have an SCI. This condition is involuntary muscle contraction distal to the level of the injury that is caused by poor communication among the brain and spinal cord. Spasticity levels grow during the initial 6 months following the injury and begin to taper off in about 12 months. Spasticity can be beneficial to assist the client in muscle preservation and improving blood perfusion, both of which can limit the development of pressure sores. Acute increases in spasticity could be a sign of a more serious condition such as skin compromise, broken bones, and bladder infections (Pedretti et al., 2018).

Heterotrophic ossification is bone that is produced in places where it should not be located. Many times, these abnormal bone growths develop around the hip muscles and knees but have also been identified in the elbow and shoulder (Kirshblum et al., 2007). Clinical symptoms appear such as inflammation and decreased ROM (Kirshblum et al., 2007). The intervention begins by sustaining a neutral pelvic position (Kedlaya, 2015). Heterotrophic ossification can lead to other positioning deficits such as scoliosis, kyphosis, and decreased skin integrity.

Sexual Abnormalities

Sexual pleasure is not affected by SCI. Deficits in functional mobility and independence, changes in body image in addition to other medical complications, partner's attitude toward people who have an SCI affect sexual roles, interest, and general satisfaction. Sensory deficits also affect sexual satisfaction. For a client to enjoy sexual intercourse they must concentrate on sensations that remain intact to experience maximum pleasure. Men frequently experience ejaculation and erection difficulties and must be remedied individually. Often sperm mobility is reduced. Women will experience menstrual dysfunction with irregular periods. Women experience vaginal dryness during sexual intercourse and fertility remains intact. Women can give birth. Contraceptives can increase the risk for women to have blood clots and diaphragms are not recommended secondary to sensation deficits. Condoms are the most reliable method of contraception (Consortium for Spinal Cord Medicine, 2010; Pregnancy and Spinal Cord Injury, 2015).

OT Intervention

Occupational therapy intervention begins with establishing the occupational profile, goals, and specific information related to the client. Discharge planning begins early in the assessment process to aid with intervention planning. The top-down approach begins with the client's symptoms and is the most common approach used to treat SCI. Occupational therapists should examine psychosocial changes due to disability and quality of life. Client motivation, attitude, and environment affect how rehabilitation will improve or limit progress. Other considerations include finances, education, social support, attitudes, and problem-solving.

ROM must be examined first and then MMT to assess if pain or contractures are present. People who have suffered C4–C7 tetraplegia usually present with shoulder pain and limited ROM. Assess sensation for light touch, superficial pain, and kinesthesia. Cognition and visual perception function should also be assessed during the acute phase of the SCI.

ADL assessment will begin as soon as the client has been released from bed rest by a physician. During the acute phase the goal is positioning, stability, and immobilization. During the active phase the goal is mobility, out of bed positioning, sitting balance, and pressure reduction.

References

Consortium for Spinal Cord Injury. (1997). *Autonomic dysreflexia: What you should know—a guide for people with spinal cord injury.* http://www.pva.org/atf/cf/{ca2a0ffb-6859-4bc1-bc96-6b57f57f0391}/consumer%20guide_autonomic%20 dysreflexia.pdf

Consortium for Spinal Cord Medicine. (2008). Early acute management in adults with spinal cord injury: A clinical practice guideline for health-care professionals. *Journal of Spinal Cord Medicine, 31,* 403–479.

Consortium for Spinal Cord Medicine. (2010). *Sexuality and reproductive health in adults with spinal cord injury: A clinical practice guideline for health-care professionals.* http://www.pva.org/atf/cf/{ca2a0ffb-6859-4bc1-bc96-6b57f57f0391} /cpg_sexuality%20and%20reproductive%20health.pdf

Ditunno, J., Cardenas, D., Formal, C., & Dalal, K. (2012). Advances in the rehabilitation management of acute spinal cord injury. *Handbook of Clinical Neurology, 109,* 181–195.

Grant, R., Quon, J., & Abbed, K. (2015). Management of acute traumatic spinal cord injury. *Current Treatment Options in Neurology, 17,* 1–13. doi:10.1007/s11940-014-0334-1

Juknis, N., Cooper, J., & Volshteyn, O. (2012). The changing landscape of spinal cord injury. *Handbook of Clinical Neurology, 109,* 149–166.

Kedlaya, D. (2015). *Heterotopic ossification in spinal cord injury.* http://emedicine.medscape.com/article/322003-overview#a1

Kirshblum, S., Priebe, M. M., Ho, C. H., Scelza, W. M., Chiodo, A. E., & Wuermser, L.-A. (2007). Spinal cord injury medicine. Part 3. Rehabilitation phase after acute spinal cord injury. *Archives of Physical Medicine and Rehabilitation, 88,* S62–S70. doi:10.1016/j.apmr.2006.12.003

Kirshblum, S., Botticello, A., Lammertse, D. P., Marino, R. J., Chiodo, A. E., & Jha, A. (2011). The impact of sacral sensory sparing in motor complete spinal cord injury. *Archives of Physical Medicine and Rehabilitation, 92,* 376–383. doi:10.1016/japmr.2010.07.242

McKinley, W., Santos, K., Meade, M., & Brooke, K. (2007). Incidence and outcomes of spinal cord injury clinical syndromes. *Journal of Spinal Cord Medicine, 30,* 215–224.

Model Systems Knowledge Translation Center. (2011). *Spasticity and spinal cord injury.* http://www.msktc.org/lib/docs /factsheets/sci_spasticity_and_sci.pdf

National Institute of Neurological Disorders and Stroke. (2014). *NINDS central cord information page.* https://www.sci -info-pages.com/wp-content/media/SCI-Spasticity.pdf

Pedretti, L. W., Pendleton, H. M. H., & Schultz-Krohn, W. (2018). *Pedretti's occupational therapy: Practice skills for physical dysfunction* (8th ed.). Elsevier.

Pregnancy and spinal cord injury (2015). http://sexualhealth.sci-bc.ca/scipregnancy/

Roberts, T. T., Leonard, G. R., & Cepela, D. J. (2017). Classifications in brief: American Spinal Injury Association (ASIA) Impairment Scale. *Clinical Orthopaedics and Related Research, 475*(5), 1499–1504. https://doi.org/10.1007/ s11999-016-5133-4

CPSIA information can be obtained
at www.ICGtesting.com
Printed in the USA
LVHW051252040821
694271LV00001B/1